T0075233

ENT Vivas

This clear and concise text covers all the assessable aspects of the ENT curriculum for the FRCS. Although technique and presentation of knowledge will no doubt be attained through viva practice, the comprehensive content ensures that all candidates have the relevant knowledge not only to succeed but also to excel in their viva examination. Covering both the theoretical and clinical aspects of the examination, as well as other equally critical aspects, including communication skills, clinical examination and miscellaneous sections, this handbook is a high-yield revision aid for all surgical trainees in the early stages of their Otolaryngology careers and simultaneously acts as an emergency information source for those cross-covering the specialty. ENT/Otorhinolaryngology surgical trainees and residents will find the scope of this guide highly relevant to obtain FRCS accreditation or equivalent.

Adnan Darr is currently an advanced rhinology and skull base fellow at Nottingham University Hospitals NHS Trust, having undertaken his higher surgical training within the West Midlands.

Karan Jolly has completed his higher surgical training in the West Midlands and is currently pursuing a rhinology and anterior skull base fellowship at the Vancouver General Hospital and St Paul's sinus centre in Vancouver.

Jameel Muzaffar is currently TWJ Foundation Fellow in Otology and Auditory Implantation at Cambridge University Hospitals and the Sensory Encoding and Neuro-biological Systems Engineering (SENSE) Laboratory, Department of Clinical Neurosciences at the University of Cambridge.

MasterPass Series

100 Medical Emergencies for Finals
Prasanna Sooriakumaran, Channa Jayasena, Anjla Sharman

300 Essential SBAs in Surgery: With Explanatory Answers
Kaji Sritharan, Samia Ijaz, Neil Russel

Cases for Surgical Finals: SAQs, EMQs and MCQs
Philip Stather, Helen Cheshire

Dermatology Postgraduate MCQs and Revision Notes
James Halpern

The Final FRCA Short Answer Questions: A Practical Study Guide
Elizabeth Combeer

Advanced ENT training: A guide to passing the FRCS (ORL-HNS) examination
Joseph Manjaly, Peter Kullar

The Final FRCR: Self-Assessment
Amanda Rabone, Benedict Thomson, Nicky Dineen, Vincent Helyar, Aidan Shaw

Geriatric Medicine: 300 Specialist Certificate Exam Questions
Shibley Rahman, Henry Woodford

Clinical Cases for the FRCA: Key Topics Mapped to the RCoA Curriculum
Alisha Allana

MCQs, MEQs and OSPEs in Occupational Medicine: A Revision Aid
Ken Addley

ENT Vivas: A Guide to Passing the FRCS (ORL-HNS) Viva Examination
Adnan Darr, Karan Jolly, Jameel Muzaffar

For more information about this series please visit: https://www.routledge.com/MasterPass/book-series/CRCMASPASS

ENT Vivas

A Guide to Passing the Intercollegiate FRCS (ORL-HNS) Viva Examination

Edited by

Adnan Darr
BSc (Hons), MSc, MBChB, DOHNS, PGCME, FRCS (ORL-HNS)
Advanced Rhinology & Anterior Skull Base Fellow
Nottingham University Hospitals NHS Trust,
Queens Medical Centre, Nottingham, UK

Karan Jolly
MBChB, FRCS (ORL-HNS)
Advanced Rhinology & Anterior Skull Base Fellow
University of British Columbia, Vancouver General Hospital,
Vancouver, Canada

Jameel Muzaffar
BA (Hons), MBBS (Hons), MSc, FRCS (ORL-HNS)
TWJ Foundation Otology & Auditory Implantation Fellow
Cambridge University Hospitals/University of Cambridge,
Addenbrooke's Hospital, Cambridge, UK

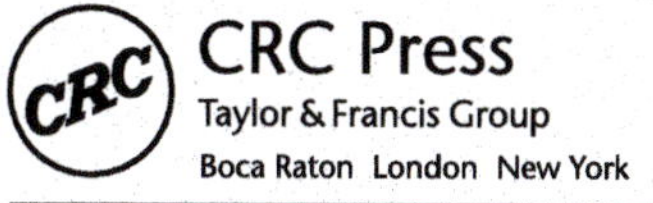

CRC Press is an imprint of the
Taylor & Francis Group, an informa business

First edition published 2023
by CRC Press
6000 Broken Sound Parkway NW, Suite 300, Boca Raton, FL 33487-2742

and by CRC Press
4 Park Square, Milton Park, Abingdon, Oxon, OX14 4RN

CRC Press is an imprint of Taylor & Francis Group, LLC

Library of Congress Cataloging-in-Publication Data

Names: Darr, Adnan, editor. | Jolly, Karan, editor. | Muzaffar, Jameel, editor.
Title: ENT vivas : a guide to passing the intercollegiate FRCS (ORL-HNS) viva examination / edited by Adnan Darr, Karan Jolly, Jameel Muzaffar.
Description: First edition. | Boca Raton : CRC Press, 2022. | Includes bibliographical references and index.
Identifiers: LCCN 2022005434 (print) | LCCN 2022005435 (ebook) | ISBN 9781032161099 (hardback) | ISBN 9781032113401 (paperback) | ISBN 9781003247098 (ebook)
Subjects: MESH: Otorhinolaryngologic Diseases | Otorhinolaryngologic Surgical Procedures--methods | Study Guide
Classification: LCC RF46 (print) | LCC RF46 (ebook) | NLM WV 18.2 | DDC 617.5/1--dc23/eng/20220624
LC record available at https://lccn.loc.gov/2022005434
LC ebook record available at https://lccn.loc.gov/2022005435

ISBN: 978-1-032-16109-9 (hbk)
ISBN: 978-1-032-11340-1 (pbk)
ISBN: 978-1-003-24709-8 (ebk)

DOI: 10.1201/9781003247098

Typeset in Adobe Garamond Pro
by KnowledgeWorks Global Ltd.

I would like to thank my wife Nadia, daughter Hanna, son Aydin, and entire family. My journey to where I am now would not have been possible without your continued support and patience, for which I will forever be indebted. To Prof Nicholas Spyrou, who is no longer with us but was the biggest influence behind my decision to pursue a career in medicine.

Adnan Darr

I dedicate this book to my wife Pawan and my parents, who have selflessly helped and allowed me to become who I am today. Your love and support will never be forgotten.

Karan Jolly

To my wife Dominique, my family, colleagues and friends. Your patience, support and understanding make everything possible.

Jameel Muzaffar

Contents

Foreword

Higher surgical exams conducted by the Royal Colleges in UK have been the gold standard in 'signing off' trainees into independent practice. It was the Royal Charter in 1843 which created the Royal College of Surgeons in England as we know it today and also created a higher qualification, the Fellowship of the College (FRCS), to recognise specialists. It took another 68 years before Eleanor Davies-Colley became the first female Fellow in 1911. It quickly became the benchmark qualification for higher surgical training across the globe. The current intercollegiate exams in Otolaryngology replaced the 'old style FRCS' in 1996 as the 'exit exam' leading towards Certificate of Completion of Training (CCT) and specialist registration with the General Medical Council.

For trainees planning to undertake this exam, it is essential to take it only when fully prepared for it. It is fundamentally an exam which tests their knowledge as they apply it in their everyday clinical practice, designed at the level of a 'day-one' consultant. The editors of this book—Adnan Darr, Karan Jolly, Jameel Muzaffar—and the various contributors have produced a resource to add to the list of books which will help prepare trainees for exit exams all over the world. I would like to congratulate them on this endeavour and their efforts to help junior colleagues to progress in their careers.

Professor M Shahed Quraishi, OBE, FRCS, FRCSEd, FRCS (ORL-HNS)
Consultant Otolaryngologist, Thyroid and Parathyroid Surgeon, Doncaster Royal Infirmary
President, Royal Society of Medicine 2018-19 (Laryngology & Rhinology Section)
Director, ENT Masterclass®
Visiting Professor Capital Medical University, Beijing
Hon Senior Lecturer in Surgical Oncology, University of Sheffield

Preface

The Intercollegiate Fellowship in Otorhinolaryngology (FRCS [ORL-HNS]) is a key milestone in the training of Ear, Nose and Throat surgeons in the United Kingdom and elsewhere. It represents the most significant hurdle to overcome in the latter stages of training and exam success often marks a shift in confidence of successful candidates, with many reporting that they felt a change in their interactions with consultant trainers as well as enjoying informal approaches regarding potential consultant jobs. All of this is of limited comfort to those setting out on the road to exam success. The authors recognise the pressure that comes with the peri-exam period. We all vividly remember the feelings of not having enough time to master the insurmountable volume of content, the nagging feeling that you should be working during any downtime from studying and the resentment at the time spent away from friends and family whilst preparing for the exam.

A significant challenge for any exam candidate is finding texts pitched at the level of the exam with concise summaries and key points. We hope that this text will be of benefit to you both as a study aid for longer periods and also during breaks between theatre cases or in some of the other pockets of dead time we can all make better use of. A key aspect of success, particularly in Part II of the exam, is being able to present your knowledge in a structured and coherent way. Each topic follows the same format to facilitate recall and ensure that you have command of key aspects of each presentation. Topics have been written by early stage consultants, post-CCT fellows or exceptional registrars near the end of training.

We hope that you find the text valuable and would love to hear your thoughts, whether this was the case or you have suggestions for improvement.

Adnan Darr, Karan Jolly and Jameel Muzaffar
Nottingham, Vancouver and Cambridge, 2022

Editors

Adnan Darr is currently an advanced rhinology and skull base fellow at Nottingham University Hospitals NHS Trust, having undertaken his higher surgical training within the West Midlands. He maintains a strong passion for education, having held roles as an educational fellow and honorary clinical lecturer at the University of Birmingham, where he received a REME (Recognition of Excellence in Medical Education) award. He has held the role of national audit lead for the British Rhinological Society Juniors (BRSJ) and has maintained an active role in research throughout his medical career. Adnan has a keen interest in endoscopic approaches to the anterior skull base, as well as advanced imaging of the head and neck, having trained as a physicist prior to a career in medicine.

Karan Jolly has completed his higher surgical training in the West Midlands and is currently pursuing a rhinology and anterior skull base fellowship at the Vancouver General Hospital and St Paul's sinus centre in Vancouver. He has a keen interest in endoscopic skull base surgery and is currently working towards a PhD in endoscopic skull base reconstruction and is the first UK trainee to have successfully completed the European diploma of endoscopic skull base surgery from Paris university. In addition to his clinical interests, he remains very active in research and education. Karan has specific interests in simulated training for rhinology and management of skull base tumours.

Jameel Muzaffar is currently TWJ Foundation Fellow in Otology and Auditory Implantation at Cambridge University Hospitals and the Sensory Encoding and Neuro-biological Systems Engineering (SENSE) Laboratory, Department of Clinical Neurosciences at the University of Cambridge. He was previously a trainee on the West Midlands Higher Surgical Training scheme, including three years of Out of Programme Research for a PhD followed by a year of split clinical and academic training. He is currently National Trainee Lead for the NIHR ENT Clinical Research Network having previously been Regional Lead for the West Midlands. Jameel is interested in most aspects of hearing health, but particularly implantable devices, tech as applied to the ear and clinical and translational research.

Contributors

Co-Authors

Paula Coyle BSc (Hons), BMBS (Hons), DOHNS, DCH, FRCS (ORL-HNS)
Senior Paediatric ENT Clinical Fellow
Great Ormond Street Hospital, Great Ormond Street, London, UK

Keshav Kumar Gupta BSc (Hons), MRCS (ENT)
ST3 ENT Registrar
Birmingham Heartlands Hospital, University Hospitals Birmingham NHS Foundation Trust, Birmingham, UK

Hannah Nieto BSc, MBBS, MRCS, FRCS (ORL-HNS), PhD
NIHR Academic Clinical Lecturer, ST7 ENT Registrar
University of Birmingham, Edgbaston, Birmingham, UK

Anna Slovick BSc (Hons), MBBS, DOHNS, FRCS (ORL-HNS)
Locum Consultant ENT Surgeon
Royal National ENT Hospital and Eastman Dental Hospitals, London, UK

Chloe Swords MA (Cantab), MBBS, MRCS (ENT)
Research Fellow and PhD Student
Department of Clinical Neurosciences, University of Cambridge, Addenbrooke's Hospital, Cambridge, UK

Theofano Tikka MBBS, MSc, MCh (ENT), MMEd, FHEA, FRCS (ORL-HNS)
ST8 ENT Registrar
Queen Elizabeth University Hospital, Glasgow, UK

Senior Editors

Manohar Bance MBChB, MSc, FRCS (ORL-HNS), FRCSC, ABOto
Professor of Otology and Skull Base Surgery
University of Cambridge/Cambridge University Hospitals, Addenbrooke's Hospital, Hills Road, Cambridge, UK

Eishaan Kamta Bhargava MBBS, MS (ENT), FRCS (ORL-HNS)
Consultant Paediatric ENT Surgeon
Sheffield Children's Hospital, Western Bank, Sheffield, UK

Sanjiv Bhimrao MBBS, MS, DM, FRCS (ORL-HNS)
Consultant ENT Surgeon
University Hospitals of North Midlands NHS Trust, Royal Stoke University Hospital, Stoke-on-Trent, UK

Wai Sum Cho BMedSci, BMBS, FRCS (ORL-HNS)
Locum Consultant ENT Surgeon
Nottingham University Hospitals NHS Trust, Queens Medical Centre, Nottingham, UK

Claire Hopkins BMBCH, BA, Doctorate of Medicine, FRCS (ORL-HNS)
Consultant ENT Surgeon and Professor of Rhinology
Guy's and St Thomas' NHS Foundation Trust, Great Maze Pond, London, UK

Michael Kuo MBChB, FRCS (Eng), FRCS (ORL-HNS), PhD, DCH
Consultant Paediatric ENT Surgeon
Birmingham Children's Hospital, Birmingham, UK

Vinidh Paleri, MBBS, MS (ENT), FRCS (Glas), FRCS (Eng), FRCS (ORL-HNS)
Professor of Head and Neck Surgery
The Royal Marsden NHS Foundation Trust, London, UK
Institute of Cancer Research, London UK

Paul Pracy BSc, MBBS, FRCS Glas (Gen Surg), FRCS (ENT), FRCS ORL-HNS
Consultant Head and Neck Surgeon
University Hospitals Birmingham NHS Foundation Trust, Birmingham UK

Kate Stephenson FRCS (ORL-HNS [Eng]), FC ORL (SA), MMed
Consultant Paediatric ENT Surgeon
Birmingham Children's Hospital, Birmingham, UK

List of Abbreviations

AA	Atlanto-axial
AB word score	Arthur Boothroyd word score
ABG	Air Bone Gap
ABI	Auditory Brainstem Implant
ABR	Auditory Brainstem Response
ACE	Angiotensin Converting Enzyme
ACHA	Air conduction hearing aid
ACTH	Adrenocorticotropic hormone
AEA	Anterior Ethmoidal Artery
AFP	Alpha-Fetoprotein
AFS	Allergic Fungal Sinusitis
AIHL	Autoimmune Hearing Loss
ALT flap	Anterolateral thigh flap
ANA	Antinuclear Antibody
ANCA	Antineutrophil Cytoplasmic Antibodies
ANS	Anterior Nasal Spine
Anti-CCP	Anti-Cyclic Citrullinated Peptide test
AOAE	Automated Otoacoustic Emission
AOM	Acute Otitis Media
APA	Ascending Pharyngeal Artery
APD	Afferent Pupillary Defect
APGAR	Appearance, Pulse, Grimace, Activity and Respiration
APLS	Advanced Paediatric Life Support
ARIA	Allergy and Rhinitis in Asthma
ARS	Allergic Rhinosinusitis
ASD	Atrial Septal Defect
ASHA	American Speech Language Hearing Association
Association	Multiple congenital anomalies occurring at high frequency together
ATLS	Advanced Trauma Life Support
AVM	Arteriovenous Malformation
BAER	Brainstem Auditory Evoked Response
BAETS	The British Association of Endocrine and Thyroid Surgeons

BAHA	Bone Anchored Hearing Aid
BAHI	Bone Anchored Hearing Instrument
BAHS	Bone Anchored Hearing System
BBB	Blood Brain Barrier
BC	Bone Conduction
BCC	Basal Cell Carcinoma
BCHA	Bone Conduction Hearing Aid
BEA	Behind the Ear (hearing) Aid
BiCROS	Bilateral microphones with Contralateral Routing Of Signal
BIH	Benign Intracranial Hypertension
BKB	Bamford-Kowal-Bench sentence test
BM	Boehringer Mannheim (a commonly used test for blood sugar monitoring)
BMI	Body Mass Index
BORS	Branchio-Oto-Renal Syndrome
Ca	Calcium
CAT	Combined Approach Tympanoplasty
CBT	Cognitive Behavioural Therapy
CCF	Congestive Cardiac Failure
CFTR	Cystic Fibrosis Transmembrane Conductance Regulator
CHARGE	Coloboma, Heart, Atresia of choanae, Retardation of growth and development, Genital and urinary anomalies and Ear abnormalities
CHD	Coronary Heart Disease
CHL	Conductive hearing Loss
CI	Cochlear Implant
Cis	Carcinoma in situ
CLD	Chronic Lung Disease
cm	Centimetre
CMV	Cytomegalovirus
CN	Cranial Nerve
CNS	Clinical Nurse Specialist
CNS	Central Nervous System
CNVII	Cranial Nerve VII (Facial Nerve)
CNVIII	Cranial Nerve VIII (Auditory Nerve)
CO	Carbon Monoxide
CO2	Carbon Dioxide
COPD	Chronic Obstructive Pulmonary Disease
CPA	Cerebellopontine Angle
CPAP	Continuous Positive Airway Pressure
CROS	Contralateral Routing of Signal
CRP	C-Reactive Protein
CRS	Chronic Rhinosinusitis

CRT	Chemoradiotherapy
CSF	Cerebrospinal Fluid
CSOM	Chronic Suppurative Otitis Media
CST	Cavernous Sinus Thrombosis
CT	Chemotherapy
CT	Computerised Tomography
CV	Cardiovascular
CVA	Cerebrovascular Accident (Stroke)
CVS	Cardiovascular System
CVST	Cerebral Venous Sinus Thrombosis
CWD	Canal Wall Down
CWU	Canal Wall Up
CXR	Chest X-ray
dB A	Decibel (A weighted)
dB C	Decibel (C weighted)
dB HL	Decibel Hearing Level
DCR	Dacrocystorhinostomy
DH	Drug history
DIC	Disseminated Intravascular Coagulation
DM	Diabetes Mellitus
DPOAE	Distortion Product Otoacoustic Emission
DsDNA	Double stranded DNA
DTPA	Diethylenetriamine Pentaacetate
DVT	Deep Vein Thrombosis
DWI	Diffusion Weighted Imaging (type of MRI)
EAC	External Auditory Canal
EBRT	External beam radiotherapy
EBV	Epstein-Barr Virus
ECA	External Carotid Artery
ECG	Electrocardiogram
ECS	Extracapsular spread
EEG	Electroencephalography
eGFR	Estimated glomerular filtration rate
EMG	Electromyogram
ENoG	Electroneurography
EOG	Electrooculogram
ESR	Erythrocyte Sedimentation Rate
ESS	Endoscopic Sinus Surgery
ET	Endotracheal Tube
ETD	Eustachian Tube Dysfunction
EUA	Examination under Anaesthetic
FB	Foreign Body
FBC	Full Blood Count

FEES	Fiberoptic Endoscopic Evaluation of Swallowing
FESS	Functional Endoscopic Sinus Surgery
FFP	Fresh Frozen Plasma
FH	Family History
FNAC	Fine Needle Aspiration Cytology
FNE	Fibreoptic Nasendoscopy
Ga	Gadolinium (contrast for MRI)
GBS	Guillain-Barré syndrome
GCS	Glasgow Coma Score
GI	Gastrointestinal
GORD	Gastro-Oesophageal Reflux Disease
GPA	Granulomatosis with Polyangiitis
GSPN	Greater Superficial Petrosal Nerve
HA	Hearing Aid
HbA1C	Glycated haemoglobin
HBO	Hyperbaric Oxygen
HCG	Human Chorionic Gonadotropin
HDU	High Dependency Unit
HFA	High Frequency Average
HFHL	High Frequency Hearing Loss
HHT	Hereditary Haemorrhagic Telangiectasia
HiB	Haemophilus Influenzae Type B
HIV	Human Immunodeficiency Virus
HL	Hearing Loss
HME	Heat Moisture Exchange
HNCSCC	Head and neck squamous cell cancer
HPV	Human papilloma virus
HRCT	High Resolution CT
HSV	Herpes Simplex Virus
HTN	Hypertension
I131	Radioactive iodine
IAC	Internal Auditory Canal
IAM	Internal Acoustic Meatus
IC	Intercostal
ICA	Internal Carotid Artery
ICP	Intracranial Pressure
Ig	Immunoglobulin
IgM	Immunoglobulin M
IHC	Inner Hair Cell
IHD	Ischaemic Heart Disease
IIH	Idiopathic Intracranial Hypertension
IJV	Internal jugular vein
IMRT	Intensity modulated radiotherapy

IOP	Intraocular Pressure
IT	Intratympanic
ITSI	Intratympanic Steroid Injection
ITU	Intensive Care Unit
IV	Intravenous
JIA	Juvenile Idiopathic Angiofibroma
JNA	Juvenile Nasopharyngeal Angiofibroma
JV	Jugular Vein
kHz	kilohertz
KTP	Potassium Titanyl Phosphate
LA	Local Anaesthetic
LASER	Light Amplification by Stimulated Emission of Radiation
LDH	Lactate dehydrogenase
LFTs	Liver Function Tests
LL	Left lower
LME	Lines of Maximal Extensibility
LMN	Lower Motor Neuron
LPR	Laryngopharyngeal reflux
LSCC	Lateral Semicircular Canal
Lt	Left
LTB	Laryngotracheobronchoscopy
LTR	Laryngeal tracheal Reconstruction
MALT	Mucosa associated lymphoid tissue
MC&S	Microscopy Cultures and Sensitivities
MDT	Multidisciplinary Team
MEI	Middle Ear Implant
MEN	Multiple endocrine neoplasia
Mg	Magnesium
MG	Myasthenia Gravis
MHL	Mixed Hearing Loss
MLB	Microlaryngoscopy and Bronchoscopy
MMA	Middle Meatal Antrostomy
MMF	Maxillomandibular Fixation
MOE	Malignant Otitis Externa
MPO	Myeloperoxidase
MRA	Magnetic Resonance Angiography
MRI	Magnetic Resonance Imaging
MRND	Modified radical neck dissection
MRV	Magnetic Resonance Venography
MS	Multiple sclerosis
MSK	Musculoskeletal
MST	Maximal Stimulation Test
N staging	Nodal staging

NCS	Nerve Conduction Studies
ND	Neck dissection
NET	Nerve Excitability Test
NF	Neurofibromatosis
NF2	Neurofibromatosis Type 2
NICU	Neonatal Intensive Care Unit
NOHL	Non-Organic Hearing Loss
non-EPI	Non Echo Planar Imaging (type of MRI)
NSAID	Non-Steroidal Anti Inflammatory Drug
OAE	Oto-Acoustic Emission
OC	Ossicular Chain
OCR	Ossicular Chain Reconstruction
OD	Once daily
OE	Otitis Externa
OGD	Oesophago-gastro-duodenoscopy
OHC	Outer Hair Cell
OME	Otitis media with effusion
ORIF	Open Reduction Internal Fixation
OSA	Obstructive sleep apnoea
PALS	Patient Advice and Liaison Service
PAN	Polyarteritis Nodosa
PCD	Primary Ciliary Dyskinesia
PDA	Patent Ductus Arteriosus
PEA	Posterior Ethmoidal Artery
PES	Pharyngo-oesophageal segment
PET	Positron emission tomography
PFAPA	Periodic Fever, Aphthous Stomatitis, Pharyngitis, Adenitis
PICU	Paediatric Intensive Care Unit
PMH	Past Medical History
PN	Perineural
PND	Postnasal Drip
PNS	Postnasal Space
PO	Per Os (Latin for "by mouth")
PORP	Partial Ossicular Replacement Prosthesis
PORT	Post-operative radiotherapy
PPI	Proton Pump Inhibitor
PR3	Proteinase-3
PRS	Pierre Robin Sequence
PT	Parathyroid
PTA	Pure Tone Audiogram
PTH	Parathyroid Hormone
PTU	Propylthiouracil
PUD	Peptic Ulcer Disease
QDS	Four times daily

QoL	Quality of Life
RA	Rheumatoid arthritis
RCC	Red Cell Concentrate
RF	Rheumatoid factor
RF	Rheumatoid Factor
RF energy	Radiofrequency
RLN	Recurrent laryngeal nerve
RSTL	Relaxed Skin Tension Lines
RSV	Respiratory Syncytial Virus
Rt	Right
RT	Radiotherapy
RTA	Road Traffic Accident
SALT	Speech and Language Therapy
SC	Subcostal
SCBU	Special Care Baby Unity
SCC	Squamous cell carcinoma
SCM	Sternocleidomastoid muscle
SE	Side effects
Sequence	Group of structural abnormalities as a result of one major anomaly
SGL	Supraglottic laryngeal cancer
SIGN	Scottish Intercollegiate Guidelines Network
SLE	Systemic Lupus Erythematosus
SLN	Superior laryngeal nerve
SMG	Submandibular gland
SND	Selective neck dissection
SNHL	Sensorineural Hearing Loss
SNUC	Sinonasal Undifferentiated Carcinoma
SOB	Shortness of breath
SPA	Sphenopalatine Artery
SPF	Sphenopalatine Foramen
SPL	Sound Pressure Level
SSNHL	Sudden Sensorineural Hearing Loss
STA	Superior Thyroid Artery
STIR	Short T1 inversion recovery
STSG	Split Thickness Skin Graft
SV	Stria Vascularis
Syndrome	Group of symptoms or predictable combination of anomalies for which an identifiable cause is not necessarily understood
T staging	Tumour staging
T3	Triiodothyronine
T4	Thyroxine
TAOAE	Transient Evoked Otoacoustic Emissions
TB	Tuberculosis

Tc-99m	Metastable nuclear isomer of Technetium-99
TDS	Three times daily
TEOAE	Transient Evoked Otoacoustic Emission
TF	Temporalis Fascia
TFT	Thyroid Function Tests
Tg	Thyroglobulin
TGDC	Thyroglossal Duct Cyst
TH	Thyroid Hormone
TLM	Transoral Laser Microsurgery
TM	Tympanic Membrane
TMJ	Temporomandibular Joint
TOF	Tracheoesophageal Fistula
TOP	Trachea-Oesophageal Puncture
TORCH	Toxoplasmosis, Rubella, Cytomegalovirus, Herpes Simplex, HIV
TORCH	(T)oxoplasmosis, (O)ther Agents, (R)ubella (also known as German Measles), (C)ytomegalovirus, and (H)erpes Simplex
TORP	Total Ossicular Replacement Prosthesis
TORS	Transoral Robotic Surgery
TPO	Thyroid Peroxidase
TRT	Tinnitus Retraining Therapy
TSH	Thyroid stimulating hormone
TSI	Thyroid Stimulating Immunoglobulins
TVP	Tensor Veli Palatini
TXA	Tranexamic Acid
U&Es	Urea and Electrolytes
UPSIT	University of Pennsylvania Smell Identification Test
URTI	Upper Respiratory Tract Infection
USS	Ultrasound Scan
VATS	Video-Assisted Thoracoscopic Surgery
VDRL	Venereal Disease Research Laboratory test
VEGF	Vascular Endothelial Growth Factor
VF	Vocal Fold
VHI	Voice Handicap Index
VPI	Velopharyngeal Insufficiency
VRA	Visual Reinforcement Audiometry
VS	Vestibular Schwannoma
VSD	Ventricular Septal Defect
VZ	Varicella-zoster
WCC	White Cell Count
XR	X-ray

Chapter 1

Head and Neck

Hannah Nieto, Theofano Tikka, Adnan Darr, Karan Jolly, Paul Pracy and Vinidh Paleri

Contents

DOI: 10.1201/9781003247098-1

Ranula

1. Background:
   - A mucous extravasation cyst within floor of mouth, due to disruption of flow from minor, sublingual (most commonly) or salivary glands
   - Non-epithelial lined (pseudocyst), and walled off by epithelioid cells (activated macrophages and epithelioid cells)
   - Lateral location (distinguishing it from dermoid)
   - Deemed a plunging ranula if passing through mylohyoid muscle (partition of submandibular and sublingual space)
   - Secondary to outflow obstruction due to stricture formation, calculi or trauma
2. History:
   - Onset, periodicity, increase in size
   - Red flags: Dysphagia, dysphonia, dyspnoea, odynophagia
   - PMH:
     - History of salivary calculi/sialadenitis
     - Previous salivary gland surgery
     - Trauma, dental work
   - SH:
     - Smoking
     - Drinking
     - Betel nut chewing
3. Examination:
   - Head and neck examination, to assess for nodal disease in event of malignancy as well as extent (plunging)
   - Will transilluminate
   - Flexible nasolaryngoscopy
4. Investigations:
   - Usually on clinical grounds
   - MRI (T2 weighted) if diagnosis is questionable
5. Management:
   - Conservative:
     - Reserved for asymptomatic ranulas

- Medical: Antibiotics for infected ranula
- Surgical:
  - Aspiration (associated with high rates of recurrence: 80–100%), usually for symptomatic relief
  - Sclerotherapy with OK-432/Picibanil (derived from *Streptococcus pyogenes*)
  - Marsupialisation (+ packing for 7–10 days, reduces risk of recurrence to 0%) – re-epithelialise
  - Excision with sublingual gland (most commonly, but can be related to SMG) reduces recurrence (recurrence rates 0%): Usually transoral route as long as oral component is excised. Can occasionally consider transcervical
    - ■ Cervical ranula treated with the excision of oral segment as well as sublingual gland, with spontaneous resolution of cervical segment
    - ■ Care must be taken not to damage lingual nerve (below duct) and submandibular duct

6. Differential diagnoses:
   - Lymphangioma/lymphovascular malformation
   - Haemangioma
   - Dermoid (usually midline)
   - Salivary gland neoplasm:
     - Benign: Pleomorphic adenoma
     - Malignant: Adenoid cystic, acinic cell, mucoepidermoid

Eagle's Syndrome

1. Background:
   - Styloid process, stylohyoid ligament (styloid to lesser cornu of hyoid) and body of hyoid are derived from second pharyngeal arch
   - Styloid process is anteromedial to mastoid and 2–3 cm in length
   - Facial nerve posterolateral
   - Medial are great vessels and CN IX–XII. Also superior constrictor and pharyngobasilar fascia
   - Attached to:
     - Three muscles:
       - ■ Stylopharyngeus, styloglossus and stylohyoid muscles
     - Two ligaments:
       - ■ Stylohyoid and stylomandibular ligaments
   - Elongated styloid process or calcified stylohyoid ligament
   - Symptoms are thought to be related to:
     - Compression of:
       - ■ Glossopharyngeal (passing over superior pharyngeal constrictor) or trigeminal nerve
       - ■ Carotid and sympathetic plexus – Horner's symptoms

        - Inflammatory changes of stylohyoid ligament
        - Irritation of pharyngeal mucosa
        - Fracture of styloid process

2. History:
    - Throat/facial/neck pain radiating to ipsilateral ear
    - Globus sensation
    - Dysphagia, odynophagia
3. Examination:
    - Intra-oral palpation within tonsillar fossa reproduces pain
    - Must rule out underlying malignancy due to referred pain
        - Head and neck examination with flexible nasolaryngoscopy
    - Loss of superficial temporal artery pulsation on head turning
    - Neurological examination may demonstrate a Horner's syndrome due to sympathetic plexus compression
4. Investigations:
    - Lateral soft tissue XR
    - If suspecting malignancy (oropharyngeal), consider MRI neck
    - Definitive test:
        - CT scan for angulation and accurate assessment
        - LA infiltration within tonsillar fossa, with relief of symptoms
5. Management:
    - Conservative:
        - Usually for non-troublesome symptoms or high risk due to co-morbidities
    - Medical:
        - Analgesics
    - Surgical:
        - Transcervical:
            - Incision 2–3 finger breadths below angle of mandible
            - Deep fascia divided and SCM retracted posteriorly
            - Posterior belly of digastric and stylohyoid muscles identified and retracted posteroinferiorly
            - Styloid medial to muscle
            - Periosteum elevated to base and styloid excised with bone cutting scissors
            - Drain in situ
            - Layered closure
        - Transoral:
            - Through tonsillar fossa
            - Dissect through pharyngobasilar fascia and superior constrictor onto styloid
            - Palpation of styloid process and elevation of pharyngeal constrictor muscle off with Freer's elevator

    - Excision with bone cutting shears or Kerrison's instruments (amputate 2–3 cm)
6. Differential diagnoses:
   - Trigeminal neuralgia
   - Migraine
   - Arthritis
   - Oropharyngeal malignancy

Pharyngeal Pouch

1. Background:
   - Raised intra-luminal pressure due to cricopharyngeal spasm = false pulsion diverticulum (only contains mucosa and submucosa)
   - 80% found on left side
   - Three types:
     - Zenker: At Killian's dehiscence: Between cricopharyngeus and thyropharyngeus (inferior constrictor muscles) – posterior position
     - Killian-Jamieson: Between oblique and transverse fibres of cricopharyngeus (risk of damage to RLN) – anteromedial position
     - Laimer's triangle: Between cricopharyngeus and superior oesophageal muscle – posterior position
   - Risk of malignancy 0.4–1.5%
2. History:
   - Dysphagia due to pressure exerted on oesophagus posteriorly
   - Regurgitation/aspiration/choking/recurrent chest infections
   - Halitosis
   - Weight loss
   - Globus
   - Hoarseness, odynophagia: Exclude the presence of SCC in pouch
3. Examination:
   - Full head and neck examination:
     - Patient may appear cachectic
     - Neck swelling (left-sided). Boyce's sign: Gurgling on palpation of anterior neck mass
     - Nasolaryngoscopy may demonstrate pooling and cord palsy
4. Investigations:
   - Contrast swallow
   - Panendoscopy and biopsy if abrupt change in symptomology suggestive of malignancy
5. Management:
   - Conservative: Speech and language therapy (SLT), thickened/modified diet/consider nasogastric tube (NG tube) or gastrostomy
     - If medically unfit for any surgery
     - Or pouch too small to excise/staple

- Medical: PPI (laryngopharyngeal reflux [LPR] causes cricopharyngeus muscle spasm)
- Surgical:
  - Panendoscopy to rule out malignant transformation
  - Endoscopic:
    - Botox to cricopharyngeal bar
    - Stapling (if >2.5 cm) using a Weerda scope and staple gun. Excision of cricopharyngeus bar inserting staple gun upside down. Day case, low morbidity
      - Complications:
        - GA
        - Orodental trauma
        - Perforation/mediastinitis
        - Failure (10–20% for all approaches)
    - CO_2 laser/diathermy to cricopharyngeus
    - CO_2 laser if <2.5 cm
  - Open:
    - Myotomy + suspension (diverticulopexy)
    - Myotomy + excision (diverticulectomy)
      - Pouch packed with ribbon gauze and bougie inserted into oesophagus to identify cricopharyngeus
      - Left-sided collar (skin crease) incision
      - SCM delineated and retracted
      - Omohyoid identified, and divided –IJV is now visible
      - Middle thyroid vein divided, with identification of RLN
      - Thyroid cartilage rotated medially and diverticulum dissected
      - Neck is clamped and diverticulum divided, or staples are used
      - Cricopharyngeal myotomy is undertaken, otherwise high risk of recurrence
      - Precaution should be taken when performing this after stapling, as the pouch mouth may be wide
      - Neck drain
      - Post-operatively:
        - Antibiotics for 1 week
        - Nasogastric tube to remain in situ for 5–7 days
        - Contrast swallow day 5–7, and if no leak, then liquids, followed by semi-solid food the following day
        - Complications:
          - Bleeding (primary or secondary)
          - Infection
          - Scar
          - Fistula
          - Perforation: Mediastinitis

- Stricture
- Recurrence (3%)
- RLN injury

Pharyngeal Pouch Staging:

Morton		*Van Overbeek*
Small	**<2 cm**	<1 vertebral body in height
Medium	**2–4 cm**	1–3 vertebral bodies in height
Large	**>4 cm**	>3 vertebral bodies in height

Laryngopharyngeal Reflux

1. Background:
   - Reflux of stomach contents into larynx and pharynx
   - Multi-factorial (with gastro-oesophageal reflux association)
   - Can remain symptomatic despite optimal reflux therapy
   - Mucosal irritation secondary to pepsin, proteolytic enzymes, bacteria and bile salts
     - Pepsin may damage extra-gastric tissues with a pH of up to 6, hence PPI therapy may not halt mucosal damage
   - Implicated in:
     - Subglottic stenosis
     - Vocal cord nodules
     - Laryngeal SCC
     - Mucosal ulcers
2. History:
   - Cough
   - Sore throat
   - Globus pharyngeus
   - Dysphonia (worse in morning)
   - Post-nasal drip, excessive mucous clearing
   - Red flags: True dysphagia, odynophagia, referred otalgia
   - PMH: Gastro-oesophageal reflux
   - DH: NSAIDs
   - SH: Smoking, alcohol
3. Examination:
   - Exclusion of upper-aerodigestive tract malignancy
   - Oropharyngeal examination to assess for tonsillar pathology (±palpation of tongue base)

- Head and neck examination: Assessment of lymphadenopathy
- Nasolaryngoscopy: Assessment of nasopharynx and larynx:
  - Inter-arytenoid oedema
  - Posterior commissure hypertrophy
  - Hyperaemic or oedematous vocal cords
  - Obliteration of laryngeal ventricle
  - Granulations of the vocal fold process
  - Subglottic oedema

4. Investigations:
   - Overnight pH monitoring (up to 80% sensitivity) or manometry (to assess lower oesophageal sphincter tone)
   - Barium swallow: Will demonstrate dysmotility, achalasia, a hiatus hernia, reflux, cricopharyngeal spasm or stricture
     - Overall yield is low, consider after malignant pathology excluded
   - Helicobacter pylori test for refractory gastro-oesophageal reflux symptoms
   - In the presence of red flags (dysphagia, otalgia, well-localised odynophagia), or features consistent with an oropharyngeal malignancy, consider panendoscopy and biopsy (or an MRI scan)
5. Management:
   - Conservative:
     - Lifestyle modifications:
       - Smoking cessation
       - Dietary alterations (avoid caffeine and alcohol, low fat and low sugar content)
       - Weight loss, avoid overeating
       - Head elevation overnight and earlier meal before bed
   - Medical:
     - Alginate such as Gaviscon Advance after meals and before bed
     - Recent RCT showing no benefit for PPI treatment
   - Follow-up in 6 weeks:
     - If no improvement and persistent symptoms, consider:
       - Transnasal oesophagoscopy if available
       - Imaging followed by endoscopic assessment, particularly for well-localised symptoms
       - OGD if associated with gastro-oesophageal reflux symptoms
   - Surgical:
     - Consider referral for consideration of fundoplication if severe associated gastro-oesophageal reflux (increases tone of distal oesophageal sphincter)
6. Differential diagnoses:
   - Exclusion of malignancy is key, and if examination findings are positive or there are significant red flags in the patient history, imaging and appropriate endoscopic assessment should be performed

7. Evidence:
   - See O'Hara J et al. Use of proton pump inhibitors to treat persistent throat symptoms: multicentre, double blind, randomised, placebo-controlled trial. BMJ 2021; 372: 4903
     - RCT of lansoprazole vs placebo for patients with a high reflux symptom index (RSI) without heartburn score – the trial results showed no treatment benefit at 16 weeks and 12 months

Laryngocoele

1. Background:
   - Air-filled dilation of the appendix (saccule) of the ventricle, communicating with laryngeal lumen
   - M>F, commonly presenting in sixth decade
   - Pathophysiology:
     - Congenital
     - Acquired: Secondary to raised intra-luminal pressure in saccule (e.g. brass instrument players or glass blowers) or associated with a malignancy
   - Can become infected generating a laryngopyocele
   - Categorised as:
     - Internal: Within laryngeal cartilage framework – less common. Fullness of false cords
     - External: Sac protrudes through thyrohyoid membrane and presents as a neck lump
     - Mixed
   - Can cause airway obstruction
2. History:
   - Cough, globus pharyngeus, fluctuating neck mass, airway compromise
   - Compression causes exertional dyspnoea or dysphagia
   - Red flags include dysphonia, odynophagia and referred otalgia
   - PMH: Chronic cough, smoking, alcohol, occupation
3. Examination:
   - Oropharyngeal examination
   - Head and neck examination: Lateral neck mass, compressible (Bryce's sign: Hissing or gurgling on compression)
   - Nasolaryngoscopy:
     - Assessment of internal component/supraglottic swelling
     - Assess for malignancy
4. Investigations:
   - CT neck: Air- or fluid-filled sac communicating with laryngeal ventricle
   - MRI: For soft tissue delineation if diagnosis uncertain

5. Management:
   - Internal: Endoscopic marsupialisation or excision (CO_2 laser):
     - Incise between aryepiglottic fold and false cord over lesion, with the aim to avoid rupture of the cyst and excise it whole
   - External or mixed: Transcervical approach
     - Transcervical skin crease incision over region of thyrohyoid membrane
     - Subplatysmal flaps raised
     - Identification and preservation of superior laryngeal nerve
     - Medialise (or divide) strap muscles
     - The laryngocele will be visible and can be delivered, the carotid sheath will be posterior
     - After dissection out and excision of the laryngocoele from the thyroid cartilage, the dehiscence in the thyrohyoid membrane can be closed
     - Direct laryngoscopy should be performed to exclude malignancy
6. Differential diagnoses:
   - Saccular cyst: Mucus-filled cyst in laryngeal ventricle, but does not communicate with the laryngeal lumen

Vocal Cord Granuloma

1. Background:
   - Layers of vocal cord:
     - Epithelium (stratified squamous, non-keratinised)
     - Superficial layer of lamina propria (Reinke's space)
     - Intermediate and deep layer of lamina propria (vocal ligament)
     - Vocalis muscle (thyroarytenoid)
   - Perichondrial inflammation of exposed cartilaginous vocal process secondary to repeated trauma
     - Phonotrauma
     - Intubation
     - Precipitated by LPR
     - Persistent cough
   - May be idiopathic
   - Usually unilateral
2. History:
   - Dysphonia: Duration and severity
   - Globus
   - PMH:
     - History of intubation
     - GORD

- SH:
  - Phonotrauma based on occupation
  - Smoking, predominantly to include/exclude malignancy as differential
  - URTI, coughing

3. Examination:
   - Full head and neck examination to rule out malignancy/metastatic disease
   - Flexible nasolaryngoscopy:
     - Posterior lesion, smooth, over vocal process
4. Investigations:
   - Biopsy to rule out malignancy
5. Management:
   - Conservative:
     - Vocal hygiene
     - SALT review for voice therapy
   - Medical:
     - PPI therapy and alginates for LPR
     - Lifestyle (positioning in bed, diet, smoking cessation, reduce alcohol)
     - Steroid inhalers
   - Surgical:
     - Intralesional steroids
     - Botox to paralyse ipsilateral cord to aid healing through reduction of contact/friction (aspiration risk, hence controversial)
       - To lateral cricoarytenoid and thyroarytenoid
     - Microlaryngoscopy + excision
       - Conventional microlaryngoscopy instruments. As a last option when above treatment options have failed, or for very large lesions.
     - Post-op voice rest for 48–72 hours
6. Differential diagnoses:
   - SCC: See handout
   - Papilloma: See relevant chapter
   - Nodules: Junction between anterior and middle 1/3 of cord due to strain, and common in singers. Bilateral. Treatment is voice therapy
   - Intracordal cyst: Usually smooth outline, with no overt features of malignancy. Investigate with stroboscopy in MDT setting. Conservative management or excision with microflap preserving medial flap but risk of sulcus vocalis
   - Polyp: Either haemorrhagic or inflammatory, with treatment similar to cyst. CO_2 laser to feeding vessel or steroid injection is also an option
   - Reinke's: More common in females, smokers. Also seen with hypothyroidism and LPR. Conservative first-line treatment (smoking cessation and voice therapy)
     - Surgery would require biopsy to exclude dysplasia/malignancy, with lateral cordotomy and aspiration

    - Reinke's is not a risk factor for malignancy, hence only biopsy if no improvement or suspicious lesions
    - SALT, smoking cessation
  - Cavernous haemangioma
  - Posterior vocal cord ulceration: TB
  - Granular cell tumour: 3% malignant

Vocal Cord Palsy

1. Background:
   - Hypotheses:
     - Semon's law: Abductors affected before adductors, hence will lie in an adducted position, hence stridor (largely historic theory)
     - Wagner-Grossman: SLN is intact so will apply an adducted force
   - Positions: Median, paramedian, intermediate (cadaveric = RLN and SLN paralysis), partial adduction, fully adducted
   - More common on left due to intrathoracic trajectory of recurrent nerve compared to right
   - Most common cause is trauma/iatrogenic. Always consider malignant disease
   - Recovery rates for idiopathic RLN palsy is 20–40%
2. History:
   - Dysphonia
   - Odynophagia, dysphagia, weight loss
   - Aspiration/recurrent chest infections, choking
   - PMH:
     - Lung cancer, lymphoma
     - Previous lung, mediastinal or neck surgery/treatment
     - Trauma to chest
     - Systemic conditions: RA can result in cricoarytenoid joint fixation (bilateral), SLE, diabetes
     - Cardiovascular
     - Neurological (usually bilateral): Parkinson's disease
     - Infections: Syphilis, Lyme disease, URTI
   - SH: Smoking
3. Examination:
   - Videostroboscopy: Jitter (frequency) and shimmer (amplitude) of mucosal wave
   - Head and neck examination:
     - Evaluate for neck masses/nodal disease or previous scars from surgery
     - Full cranial nerve examination to assess for neurological cause
     - Nasolaryngoscopy: Vocal cord movement and phonatory gap, pooling of saliva (hypopharynx malignancy)

4. Investigations:
   - Bloods: cANCA/pANCA, ACE, dsDNA antibodies, anti-SSA/SSB, anti-CCP, RF, ANA, ESR, CRP
   - CT base of skull-diaphragm
   - Laryngeal electromyography (EMG) to distinguish palsy from fixation (neural – paralysis, joint – fixation)
     - Myopathy: Normal frequency, low amplitude
     - Neuropathy: Low frequency, normal amplitude
   - Recovery prognosis on EMG
     - Denervation: At 3 weeks – fibrillation: Poor recovery
     - Re-innervation: Polyphasic potentials
   - Swallowing assessment (FEES, VF)
   - VHI (voice handicap index). Ten questions, and maximum score of 40 (never-always)
   - GRBAS (grade, roughness, breathiness, asthenia and strain): 0–3, mild, moderate, severe
   - Panendoscopy and joint palpation: When high suspicion, e.g. RA, intubation trauma, malignancy
5. Management:
   - Conservative:
     - If no evidence of aspiration or non-significant glottic gap
     - SALT input (head turn towards affected side to approximate cords better, exercises and dietary modifications)
     - Chin tuck to side of palsy
   - Medical:
     - Thickened diet
     - NG/PEG
   - Surgical (Figure 1.1):
     - Treatment with medialisation, indicated in patients with 1–3 mm phonatory gap. Early intervention advocated irrespective of pathology
     - Injection VC medialisation
       - GA via transoral
       - LA percutaneous
     - Type 1 Isshiki thyroplasty (e.g. silastic – can be reversed)
     - Arytenoid abduction (arytenoidopexy)
     - Laryngeal re-innervation: Ansa cervicalis to RLN
     - Long term and >12 months: Less likely to recover. Consider laryngeal EMG to assess recovery. If <12 months – attempt temporary measures first
     - For bilateral: Type 2 Isshiki lateralisation technique, tracheostomy, cordotomy, arytenoidectomy, arytenoidopexy, phrenic-PCA re-innervation

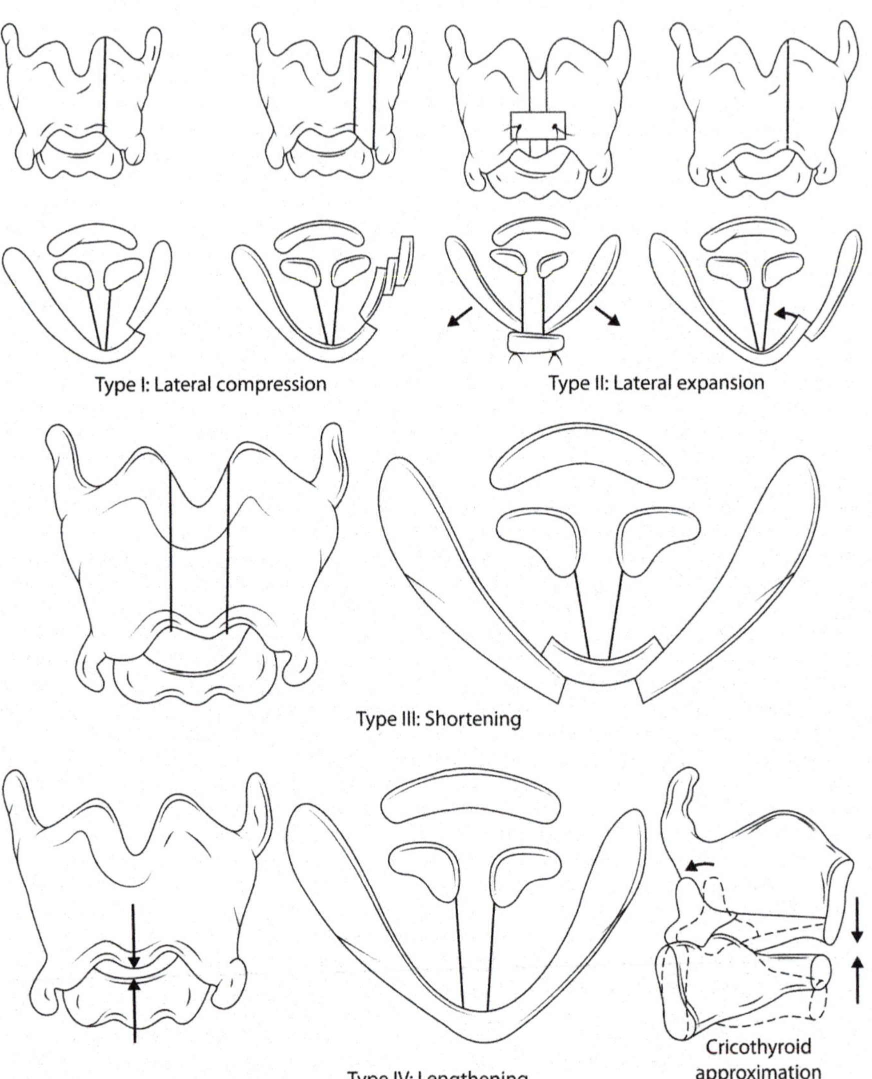

Figure 1.1 Thyroplasty types.

Causes of vocal cord immobility:

50% Iatrogenic:

- Intubation
- Thyroid surgery
- Spinal surgery
- Cardiothoracic, vascular surgery

25% Idiopathic:
- One-third full recover
- One-third partial recover
- One-third do not recover

25% Other:
- Tumours
- Neurology: Stroke, multiple sclerosis myasthenia gravis, Wallenberg syndrome
- Systemic and inflammatory: RA, SLE, sarcoidosis, diabetes (with ensuing microvascular compromise)
- Infective: Syphilis, Lyme, viral, EBV, TB
- Trauma
- Toxins

Thyroplasty types:

Type I: Medialisation, with window in thyroid cartilage, with cartilage, silastic, Gore-Tex, hydroxyapatite or titanium used for medialisation

Type II: Lateralisation, for adductor spasmodic dysphonia. Midline thyroid cartilage incision + silicon/titanium wedge used to lateralise cartilage

Type III: Relaxation for high pitch. anteroposterior shortening of thyroid ala

Type IV: Stretching/lengthening vocal cord, in patients with low pitch/bowing vocal cords (sutures between thyroid and cricoid ± plates)

Thyroplasty techniques:

- Local anaesthetic thyroplasty:
  - External approach
  - Window created within thyroid cartilage
  - Silastic block fashioned and positioned whilst position confirmed through nasolaryngoscopy
- Injection laryngoplasty:
  - Temporary:
    - Calcium hydroxyapatite (Radiesse Voice Gel), effects last from 12 months
    - Hyaluronic acid (Restylane), lasts 4–6 months
    - Gelfoam, discontinued as larger gauge needle is required
  - Permanent:
    - Teflon, now replaced due to inhibition of mucosal wave/difficulties in removal due to inflammatory reactions and granulations

  - Fat, requires harvesting from abdomen and centrifuging
    All above done either thyrohyoid, cricothyroid, transthyroid, endolaryngeal (through oropharynx) or microlaryngoscopy under general anaesthetic
- Co-Phenylcaine + nebulised Lidocaine
- Avoid injecting anterior larynx, as voice will be strained

Bilateral vocal cord fixation secondary to rheumatoid arthritis:

- Likely poorly responsive to steroids and nebulisers
- Difficult intubation:
  - C-spine immobility
  - Rigid fixed cords with nodules
  - TMJ fixation
- Management:
  - Intra-joint steroids
  - Laser cordotomy/arytenoidectomy: Poor voice/risk of aspiration
  - Arytenoidopexy: Poor voice/aspiration
  - Tracheostomy: Challenging aftercare due to poor dexterity
  - Re-innervation

Inhalational Injury

1. Background:
   - Smoke inhalation in burn patients is an independent factor in increased mortality
   - Up to 30% experience airway obstruction
   - Patients to be managed as trauma patients with assessment, and resuscitation to be performed simultaneously according to Advanced Trauma Life Support Principles (ATLS)
2. History:
   - Type of exposure: Flame, chemicals, smoke
   - Duration of exposure, exposure space
   - Loss of consciousness, other traumatic injury
   - PMH
3. Examination:
   - Airway: Stridor, dyspnoea, haemoptysis, carbonaceous sputum, singed nasal hair, mucosal ulceration
   - Breathing: Cyanosis, tachypnoea, desaturation, wheeze
   - Circulation: Hypotension, tachycardia
   - Disability: GCS (CNS depression) and irritability
   - Exposure: Other cutaneous burns

   - Remember to assess for complications/systemic toxicity, including: Pulmonary oedema, chemical tracheobronchitis, carbon monoxide poisoning
4. Investigations:
   - Arterial blood gas
     - Carboxyhaemoglobin level (>15% for admission)
       - Oxygen saturation monitoring not accurate in CO poisoning
     - PO_2 (<60 mmHg for admission)
     - Metabolic acidosis
5. Management:
   - Secure airway (can have delayed oedema)
   - Supplemental oxygen, pulmonary toilet, bronchodilators
   - No steroids
     - Doesn't improve inhalational injury and increased likelihood of infection
   - MDT management with burns team, plastics, ITU and ENT: Manage on HDU or ITU
   - Monitoring, serial arterial blood gases
   - Tracheostomy if difficult intubation or prolonged wean
   - Facial burns should be managed conservatively initially, with deep partial thickness and full thickness burns potentially needing excision of necrotic tissue at up to 10 days post-injury
   - If patients have a clinical history of potential inhalational injury but no clinical findings of such, and no cutaneous burns, they should be observed for at least 4–6 hours

Total body surface area – use the rule of 9s to calculate: Arm 9%, leg 18%, anterior and posterior trunk 18% each, head 9%, palms 1%

Parkland formula: Volume fluids per day (adults) = % total body surface area burnt × weight(kg) × 4 mL. First 8 hrs give half the volume and remaining over next 16 hrs, with strict fluid balance measurements

Blunt Laryngeal Trauma

1. Background:
   - Blunt injury is higher risk than penetrating injury for skeletal fracture
   - Paediatric fracture risk lower due to elastic cartilage but relatively high risk of soft tissue injury
   - Assess patient according to ATLS principles and secure airway early, considering the possibility of laryngotracheal separation, which can be worsened/completed by attempted endotracheal intubation
2. History:
   - Mechanism of injury: Road traffic collision, assault, clothesline
   - Dysphonia, dysphagia and odynophagia, plus possible stridor or haemoptysis

- PMH:
  - Anticoagulants
3. Examination:
   - Airway and C-spine: Stridor, dysphonia (RLN injury), haemoptysis. C-spine immobilisation in high-velocity injuries)
   - Breathing: Cyanosis, tachypnoea or desaturation due to coexisting pneumothorax/chest wall injury
   - Circulation: BP, HR
   - Disability: GCS (head injury)
   - Exposure:
     - Neck examination: Ecchymosis, range of movement, loss of laryngeal crepitus (fixation), surgical emphysema
     - Nasolaryngoscopy if within suitable environment (theatres/ED resus)
     - Assess status of larynx and classify according to Schaefer classification (Table 1.1)
     - Assess vocal cord status
     - Consider laryngotracheal separation (usually above or below the cricoid cartilage, either at the cricothyroid membrane or cricotracheal junction)

Table 1.1 Schaefer Classification System for Blunt Laryngeal Trauma

Group	*Severity/Findings*	*Management*
I	Minor endolaryngeal hematomas or lacerations without detectable fractures	Steroids Voice rest PPI, antibiotics, humidification (prevents crusting)
II	More severe oedema, hematoma, minor mucosal disruption without exposed cartilage, or non-displaced fractures	As above Direct laryngo-oesophagoscopy Serial nasolaryngoscopies
III	Massive oedema, large mucosal lacerations, exposed cartilage, displaced fractures or vocal cord immobility	Tracheostomy Direct laryngo-oesophagoscopy Repair of lacerations, VC tears, displaced cartilage through laryngofissure
IV	As group 3, but more severe with disruption of anterior larynx, unstable fractures, two or more fracture lines or severe mucosal injuries	As above Stent (ETT or glove with gelfoam): 2 weeks, removed endoscopically
V	Complete laryngotracheal separation	Secure airway. Supra and infrahyoid release and reanastomosis

4. Investigations:
   - Trauma CT series to include vertebrae and laryngeal framework
5. Management:
   - Table 1.1: Schaefer classification
   - Dislocated arytenoids require surgical intervention due to risk of crico-arytenoid fixation
   - Displaced fractures of thyroid cartilage can be managed with miniplates
6. Evidence:
   - See Moonsamy P et al. Management of laryngotracheal trauma. Ann Cardiothorac Surg. 2018; 7(2): 210–216

Penetrating Neck Trauma

1. Background:
   - Trauma generally to head and neck can be classified according to following categories:
     - High vs low velocity
     - Penetrating vs blunt
   - Low risk if platysma not breached
   - 50–70% of elective explorations are negative
   - Increased mortality in subclavian vein injury due to air embolism – midline sternotomy for repair
   - Classification by zones, see Table 1.2
2. History:
   - Mechanism of injury important (history of weapon used and ideally trajectory)
   - Symptoms by site:

Table 1.2 Zones for Penetrating Neck Trauma

Zone	*Landmarks*	*Structures at risk*
I	Clavicle (sternal notch) → cricoid (Most troublesome due to vessel retraction into mediastinum and can require thoracotomy)	Spinal cord, vertebral artery, subclavian artery, carotid artery, internal jugular vein, CNX, RLN, lung apices, brachial plexus, trachea, oesophagus, thyroid
II	Cricoid → angle of mandible	Spinal cord, vertebral artery, carotid artery, internal jugular vein, trachea, oesophagus, pharynx, CNX, RLN
III	Angle of mandible → skull base (Any vessel injury would usually require embolisation)	Spinal cord, vertebral artery, carotid artery, internal jugular vein, pharynx, sympathetic chain, CN IX–XII

Table 1.3 Hard and Soft Signs in Penetrating Neck Trauma

Soft Signs	*Hard Signs*
Dysphagia Dysphonia Non-expansile haematoma	Air bubbling/surgical emphysema Haemoptysis/haematemesis Uncontrolled bleeding Shock Expanding haematoma Neurological decline (impending CVA)

- Laryngotracheal:
  - Stridor, dyspnoea, dysphonia, haemoptysis, subcutaneous emphysema
- Oesophageal:
  - Dysphagia, odynophagia, haemoptysis, surgical emphysema: Consider bypass, or repair if <24 hrs
- Vascular injury:
  - Hypotension, tachycardia, bruit, CVA. Vertebral artery embolisation due to site and access difficulties. High mortality with carotid, but consider repair, patch, ligation

3. Examination:
   - Examine patient in safe environment (ED resus) with an ATLS approach
   - Assess for hard/soft signs, see Table 1.3
4. Investigations:
   - In those not requiring immediate surgery, and those breaching platysma, consider CT angiogram ± embolisation
   - MRI for neurological injuries
5. Management:
   - Severe injuries are managed through an MDT approach: ED, trauma, anaesthetics, orthopaedics, vascular, OMFS, general surgery
   - ATLS algorithm of ABCDE due to possibility of spinal injury
     - Airway and C-spine: C-spine immobilisation. Stridor. Secure airway through pre-existing injury if needed, or awake fibre-optic if suspected airway compromise
     - Breathing: Assess for pneumothorax/trachea injury/flail chest
     - Circulation: IV access and correct haemodynamic compromise with colloids, crystalloids or blood depending on grades of shock. Tamponade to wound. Consider Foley catheter (18–20F) or IV TXA (1 g STAT)
     - Disability: Neurological status through assessment of cranial nerves/GCS
     - Exposure:
       - Secondary survey once immediate concerns are addressed
       - Assessment of wound, possible trajectory and zones if applicable
   - Despite a normal CT angiogram, exploration may still be required if platysmal breach is seen

    - Most common vessel is IJV due to laterality
    - Carotid injury seen in 10% of cases
      - Ligation is last resort due to high risk of CVA
    - Both repaired with 6.0 prolene with cutting needle
  - Embolisation may be required for zones I and III due to difficulties with access

Facial Trauma

Nasal fractures:

1. Background:
   - Cephalic aspect thicker than the caudal end, hence cephalic fracture has higher risk of associated facial fractures
   - Rarer in children
   - Septal trauma:
     - Dislocations common where cartilage is thicker (bony-cartilage junction)
     - Fractures common where cartilage is thinner (centrally above maxillary crest)
2. Management:
   - Manipulation under local or general anaesthetic within 10–14 days, earlier in children as earlier union

Mandibular fractures:

1. Background:
   - Most common site: Condyle > angle > body > symphysis > ramus > Coronoid. But note 'U' shape of mandible creates patterns of bilateral fractures in >40% cases.
   - Coronoid protected by zygoma
   - Favourable (muscle vectors keep fractured segment in position) vs unfavourable
2. Examination:
   - Visible step in teeth or mobility of dental segments with gingival laceration
   - Sublingual haematoma considered pathognomic of anterior fracture
   - Condyle fracture with resulting shortening of mandibular height will create premature contact on the side of the fracture. i.e. patient has open bite of contralateral side
   - Trismus may be due to pain or associated zygomatic fracture impinging coronoid and temporalis muscle
3. Management:
   - Medical:
     - Prophylactic antibiotics if 'open' fracture i.e. fracture in tooth bearing region of mandible
   - Surgical:
   - Gold standard of surgical treatment <24hrs

- *Must consider favourability vs malocclusion vs patient compliance*
- Dental removal if in line of fracture or non-viable tooth
- Must consider principles of load bearing vs load sharing fixation i.e. can a mini-plate sustain the physiological forces through the mandible with the aid of fracture favourability
- ORIF standard for mandibular fractures – mini-plate place along 'ideal line of osteosynthesis' as described by Champy (load sharing fixation).
- Infected, comminuted or atrophic mandible fractures may require rigid plate fixation (load bearing)
- Condyle fractures:
  - ORIF - SORG criteria for condyle fractures – ORIF recommended if >2mm shortening or >10 degrees angulation
  - Closed reduction - Maxillomandibular fixation (MMF) archbars placed on upper and lower teeth to use elastics to guide teeth into correct occlusion – up to 6-8 weeks
- Surgical access:
  - Intra-oral (minimises damage to marginal mandibular nerve) for all simple mandibular fractures except condyle ORIF
  - External: For condyle fractures (submandibular, retromandibular, pre-auricular) (can do intra-oral endoscopic condyle ORIF) or fractures requiring extensive rigid load bearing fixation of grafting, etc.

– Complications: Lip hypoesthesia (mental nerve trauma), marginal mandibular nerve injury, non-union, malunion, TMJDS, ankylosis of TMJ, infection, osteomyelitis

Maxillary fractures:

1. Background:
   – Constitute 20% of fractures to the skull
   – Along path of least resistance
   – All involve pterygoid plates
   – Le Fort classification: Figure 1.2
     - Le Fort 1:
       - Floating palate
       - Transverse maxillary fracture
       - Upper alveolus separated from upper maxilla
       - Through anterolateral, medial maxilla and septum
     - Le Fort 2: Most common:
       - Floating maxilla (flat face)
       - Pyramidal fracture
       - Posterior alveolar ridge, through lateral wall of maxillary sinus, inferior orbital rim and nasal bones
     - Le Fort 3:
       - Floating face (craniofacial disjunction):
       - Panda facies and racoon eyes

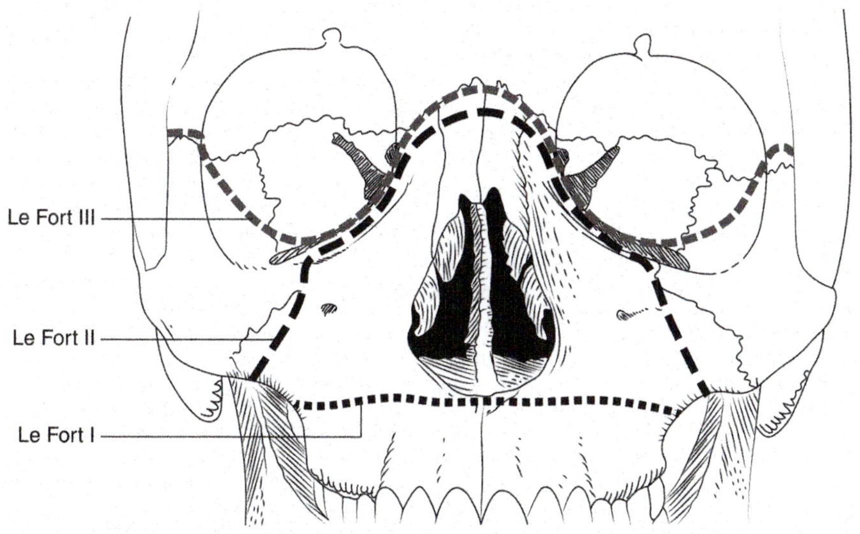

Figure 1.2 Le Fort fracture classification.

- ■ Across 3 superior suture lines
- ■ From nasofrontal suture, across maxillofrontal suture and across zygomatic arch (zygomaticofrontal suture line)

2. Management:
   - Medical: Antibiotics, analgesia
   - Surgical:
     - Immediate intervention (<24hrs) or delayed intervention (7-10 days) once oedema has resolved
     - Access: Sublabial, subciliary, degloving, coronal
     - Miniplates, intraosseus wires and bone grafts

Orbital wall fractures:

1. Background:
   - Seven bones form the orbit: Frontal, nasal, sphenoid, lacrimal, ethmoid, palatine, maxillary, zygomatic
   - Superior orbital fissure syndrome (III, IV, V1, VI)
   - Orbital apex syndrome: Optic canal (II) + superior orbital fissure syndrome (III, IV, V1, VI)
   - Blowout fractures: Are open or closed
     - Trapdoor/closed fracture: Orbital floor blowout fracture, bony segment recoils and traps orbital contents
       - ■ Mainly children (elasticity of bone) (N.B oculo-cardiac reflex causes profound bradycardia (or arrhythmia and asystole) due to intraocular muscle entrapment and vagus para n.s. stimulation, more common in children)
       - ■ Open door: Larger and displaced fractures

2. Examination:
   - Enophthalmous/hypoglobia
   - Numbness to the cheek and gums (infra-orbital nerve injury)
   - Pain, restricted eye mobility due to EOM entrapment
   - CN neuropathy:
     - CN II optic canal: Visual loss
     - CN III, IV, V1, VI (superior orbital fissure)
       - CN III: Ptosis, dilation of pupil
       - CN III, IV VI: Ophthalmoplegia
3. Management:
   - Indications for intervention:
     - Hypoglobus, enophthalmous, ophthalmoplegia, occulocardiac reflex (bradycardia), in general if defect is >50% orbital floor area then ORIF required.
   - If no occulocardiac reflex, majority of fractures treated after 7-10 days.
   - NOTE – pre-operative Orthoptic HESS chart and visual acuity assessment is mandatory before ORIF
   - Techniques:
     - Subciliary
     - Transconjunctival
     - Pre-caruncular
     - Lynch
     - Caldwell-Luc
   - ORIF implant – alloplastic (i.e, preformed titanium mesh) vs autologous (bone, cartilage or fascia)
   - Risks: Ectropian, entropian, hypoaesthesia, osteomyelitis, malunion, non-union, no improvement in symptoms

Frontal sinus fractures:

1. Background:
   - Usually resilient to trauma, thus high-velocity injuries required
   - High risk of intra-cranial involvement
   - Anterior table (12 mm) more resilient than posterior table (4 mm)
   - A third will have a CSF leak
   - A third will have anterior table fracture, but most are mixed
   - Symptoms: Swelling, pain, paraesthesia (damage to CN V_1)
   - High-resolution axial, coronal and sagittal CT scan with 3D reconstruction is the gold standard for diagnosis
2. Management:
   - Endoscopic vs open:
     - Frontal recess:
       - Obliteration
     - Anterior table fractures:

- Observation if undisplaced
- Endoscopic repair with camouflage graft is reserved for mildly displaced, in a delayed fashion
- Coronal approaches undertaken at days 7–10 and are reserved for:
  - Comminuted fractures
  - Displacement
  - Thin skin
- Posterior table fractures:
  - If undisplaced:
    - Observation if no CSF leak
    - Obliteration if CSF leak
  - If displaced:
    - Cranialisation or obliteration
- When obliterating, all remaining mucosa must be removed to minimise mucocoele formation

Examination:

Overjet:	Increased horizontal distance (jet, horizontal discrepancy)
Overbite:	Increased vertical overlap (bite down, vertical over-discrepancy)
Open bite:	Insufficient vertical overlap (vertical under-discrepancy)

Malocclusion: Angle's classification:

Class I:	Normal bite
Class II:	Retrognathia
Class III:	Prognathia

Dental classification:

Class I:	Teeth both sides of fracture
Class II:	Teeth on one side of fracture
Class III:	Edentulous

Ludwig's Angina

1. Background:
   - Life-threatening airway emergency: For assessment and resuscitation simultaneously in safe environment (ED resus or theatres)
   - Usually caused by mixed oral flora (*Staphylococcus* and *Streptococcus*)
   - Rapidly progressive cellulitis of soft tissues of floor of mouth and neck, involving collection in bilateral submandibular, submental and sublingual spaces.
   - Profound floor of mouth oedema causes displacement of the tongue and airway compromise

   - Primary site of infection is usually (90%) odontogenic, often the second or third molars (roots penetrate mylohyoid)
   - Can be precipitated by recent dental treatment, alcoholism, immunocompromise, trauma, sialadenitis and occasionally can be caused by other upper respiratory tract infections
2. History:
   - Dental history, sore throat, tonsillitis
   - Dysphagia, odynophagia, dyspnoea
   - Neck pain, trismus, drooling
   - Sepsis
   - PMH: Immunocompromise, malignancy, alcoholism
3. Examination:
   - Transfer to resus or theatres for assessment
   - Airway: Stridor
   - Breathing: Cyanosis, tachypnoea, desaturation, accessory muscle use
   - Circulation: Hypotensive and tachycardic
   - Disability: GCS, pyrexia
   - Exposure:
     - Oropharyngeal examination: Trismus, floor of mouth/posterior pharyngeal wall and peri-tonsillar region assessment
     - Head and neck examination: Torticollis, palpable firm swelling of submandibular region, associated lymphadenopathy
     - Nasolaryngoscopy: Only if deemed safe, to assess laryngeal inlet and for para and retropharyngeal swellings
4. Investigations:
   - IV access: Blood cultures, FBC, U&Es, LFTs, CRP, clotting
   - CT neck with contrast once airway secure
5. Management:
   - Secure airway
     - LA tracheostomy if required
   - Fluid resuscitation and IV antibiotics (according to trust antimicrobial guidelines, for example benzylpenicillin and metronidazole)
   - IV steroids (dexamethasone 6.6 mg)
   - Analgesia/antipyretics
   - Surgical drainage of neck abscess if present (on CT imaging)
     - Address primary source, e.g. dental abscess

Deep Space Neck Infections

1. Background:
   - Submandibular space:
     - Mylohyoid (superior), mandible (lateral), anterior belly of digastric (medial), hyoid (inferior) and muscles of tongue (posterior)

- Parapharyngeal space:
  - Skull base (superior), hyoid (inferior), pharynx (medial), parotid and mandible (lateral), pterygomandibular raphe (anterior) and cervical spine (posterior)
  - Fascia from styloid to tensor veli palatine muscle divides into two compartments:
    - Pre-styloid: Deep lobe of parotid, lymph nodes, fat, maxillary artery. Displacement of medial pharyngeal wall
    - Post-styloid: CN IX–XI, carotid sheath, sympathetic chain = T1–L2
- Retropharyngeal space:
  - Skull base (superior), buccopharyngeal fascia (anterior), alar fascia (posterior), carotid sheath (lateral), superior mediastinum (inferior)
  - Infections in children < 5 years secondary to URTI spreading to retropharyngeal nodes of Rouvière, which involute with age
  - Salivary and dental infections do not spread to retropharyngeal space
- Prevertebral space:
  - Bound superiorly by skull base, inferiorly by coccyx, anteriorly by prevertebral fascia and posteriorly by vertebral bodies
- Danger space between retropharyngeal and prevertebral spaces – extends from skull base to mediastinum
- Causes: Odontogenic in adults (mandibular molars in adults, maxillary in children) and tonsils in children
- Aerobic and anaerobic organisms, and consider actinomycosis (crosses fascial planes)
- Complications:
  - Airway obstruction
  - Sepsis, septic emboli and IJV thrombosis (Lemierre's syndrome [*Fusobacterium necrophorum*], as well as *Bacteroides*, *Streptococcus* and EBV)
  - Blowout/fistula
  - Nerve palsies
  - Mediastinitis
- Necrotising fasciitis:
  - Type I: Polymicrobial
  - Type II: Group A haemolytic streptococcus
  - Type III: Gas gangrene secondary to clostridium
  - Invades subcutaneous tissue and fascial planes, leading to ischaemia and anaesthesia
  - CT demonstrates subcutaneous emphysema
  - Treated with IV antibiotics, hyperbaric oxygen and debridement

2. History:
   - Preceding infection of upper aerodigestive tract or dental infection

- Dysphagia, odynophagia
- Systemic upset
- PMH: Dental procedures, tonsillitis, immunocompromised state (CT, HIV)
- DH: Recent antibiotics

3. Examination:
   - Transfer to resus/theatre due to imminent airway compromise
   - Airway: Assess for drooling and stridor. Secure airway if imminent compromise (awake fibre-optic intubation) or perform tracheostomy under local for large abscesses, prolonged intubation or Ludwig's angina
   - Breathing: Tachypnoea (acidosis), desaturation, cyanosis
   - Circulation: Hypotension, tachycardia, CRT
   - Disability: GCS, temperature
   - Exposure:
     - Oropharyngeal examination: Trismus, source (dental or tonsillar), floor of mouth cellulitis
     - Head and neck examination: Torticollis, restriction in mobility, swelling, erythema
     - Flexible nasolaryngoscopy if deemed safe or with anaesthetic support
4. Investigations:
   - IV access + FBC, U&Es, LFTs, CRP, INR, blood cultures
   - If stable, then CT neck and thorax with contrast
5. Management:
   - MDT approach: ENT, anaesthetics/ITU, theatres, microbiology
   - Medical: IV antibiotics according to trust antimicrobial guidelines, if surgical treatment not required long course (10/7)
   - Nebulised adrenaline and dexamethasone 6.6 mg
   - Surgical: If >2.5 cm abscess
     - Transoral approach
     - Transcervical:
       - ■ Incision anterior to SCM at level of hyoid
       - ■ Subplatysmal flaps, retraction of SCM and identification of paracarotid gutter until pus encountered
       - ■ Swab for MC&S, washout (saline) and insertion of corrugated drain (two – at superior and inferior limits)
       - ■ NGT insertion to aid feeding
       - ■ Water soluble contrast swallow after 72 hrs before NGT removal
6. Differential diagnoses:
   - Main differential to consider is source of infection as this may need operative management (e.g. dental extraction)

Non-Malignant Oral Pathology

Bullous disease:

Pemphigus vulgaris:

- Autoantibodies against intracellular adhesion proteins within epidermal cells causing fragile blisters that open easily
- Lesions in mouth (and other mucous membranes) common
- 15% mortality
- Nikolsky's sign positive: Top layer shedding of normal skin near bulla with trauma
- Management: Steroids and immunosuppression

Bullous pemphigoid:

- Autoantibodies against basement membrane (dermal-epidermal adhesion – desmosomes) causing tense blisters
- Lesions in mouth rare
- Primarily affects over 60-year-olds
- May be secondary to trauma, medication (e.g. gliptins, loop diuretics, PD-1 inhibitors and penicillins) or infection
- Management: Steroids, removal of cause

S – superficial; D – deep blisters

Oral lichen planus:

- Inflammatory condition affecting oral mucosa
- Types:
  - Reticular: Lacy white lines (Wickham's striae)
  - Erosive: Painful ulcerative lesions
  - Plaques: Similar to leukoplakia
  - Atrophic: Atrophy in centre of papule
- Most is idiopathic (autoimmune) but can be:
  - Medication induced (gold, antibiotics, NSAIDs)
  - Contact allergens (mercury, nickel, gold, resins) or spearmint toothpaste
  - Viral infection – hepatitis C
- 1% risk of malignancy
- Koebner phenomenon: Precipitated by local trauma
- Management: Oral hygiene, topical steroids, topical immunosuppressants

Aphthous ulcer:

- Painful shallow ulcers on keratinised squamous epithelium (hard palate spared)
- Lasting up to 14 days
- Erythematous halo with grey base
- Unknown aetiology, but can be related to Behcet's disease, Crohn's disease, trauma, B12 deficiency, folate deficiency, iron deficiency
- Management: Conservative

Leukoplakia:

- **Primary leukoplakia:**
  - Hyperkeratosis of stratum corneum
  - Irritation, smoking and infection are considered aetiologies
  - On examination, white patch that cannot be removed
  - 5% risk of malignancy, 30% chance if severe dysplasia
  - Management: Biopsy
- **Hairy leukoplakia:**
  - Benign hyperplasia
  - Found on lateral tongue
  - Associated with EBV
  - Management: High-dose acyclovir

Herpetic stomatitis: • Primary or secondary (reactivation of latent virus [HSV-1] in trigeminal ganglion) • Painful vesicles on oral and pharyngeal mucosa • HSV-2 associated with genital lesions • Management: Conservative, consider anti-viral therapy in primary or frequently recurrent disease (admission if immunocompromised, pregnant or severe infection/cannot swallow)	**Erythroplakia:** • Macule • Fiery red/velvet-like in texture • Risk factors include alcohol and tobacco • 50% risk of severe dysplasia or malignancy • Management: Excision if focal and small, biopsy if multifocal
Vincent's angina and acute necrotising ulcerative gingivitis (or trench mouth): • Fusobacterium sp., Treponema sp. and anaerobes (Bacteroides) • Infection of oral mucosal membranes causing painful ulceration • Vincent's angina: Tonsil and pharyngeal • ANUG: Oral mucosa alone • Sloughing of necrotic tissue, with halitosis and formation of pseudomembrane • Management: Antibiotics (metronidazole or penicillin) and chlorhexidine mouthwash	**Hairy tongue:** • Hypertrophy of filiform papillae (opposite to geographic tongue) • Colonisation with pigmented bacteria – black • Risk factors: Radiation, tobacco, abx, poor hygiene, associated with candida overgrowth • Consider whether patient is immunocompromised • Management: Oral hygiene measures
Necrotising sialometaplasia: • Benign inflammatory condition of minor salivary glands • Spontaneous ulceration of hard palate mucosa which never involves bone • Differential diagnosis is SCC • Management: Conservative after biopsy to exclude malignancy (heals within 6 weeks)	**Geographic tongue (benign migratory glossitis):** • Loss of filiform papillae leads to red atrophic areas • Migration of regions • Persists for several years • Management: Reassurance (can use topical anaesthetics if associated with burning sensation)

Sialolithiasis

1. Background:
   - 80–90% in SMG as mucous secreting
   - Definitions:
     - Sialectasis: Cystic dilatation

        - Sialosis: Asymptomatic, non-inflammatory, non-neoplastic swelling
        - Sialolithiasis: Salivary gland stones (calcium and hydroxyapatite composition)
        - Sialadenitis: Acute infection of salivary gland
    - Common organism *Staphylococcus aureus*, but also beta-haemolytic *streptococci*, *Haemophilus influenzae*
    - Medication induced in elderly causing dehydration: Anticholinergics, diuretics, antidepressants (TCA/SSRI)
2. History:
    - Timing/length of symptoms
    - Association with oral intake (pain/fluctuation in size)
    - Previous episodes
    - Red flags: Dysphagia, odynophagia, dysphonia
    - PMH: Autoimmune disease, previous H&N cancer, previous radiotherapy
    - SH: Smoking and drinking
3. Examination:
    - Head and neck examination:
        - Assessment of any nodal disease alongside mass
        - Floor of mouth examination (bimanual palpation)
        - Flexible nasolaryngoscopy
4. Investigations:
    - USS neck:
        - Most accessible
        - Will identify parenchymal lesions
        - May miss stricture/small calculi
    - Sialography: Second line and gold standard:
        - Will detect intra-ductal pathology
        - Small calculi may be flushed
        - Will require cannulation, which may aid flow
    - Sialendoscopy/interventional (see ahead in the chapter)
    - MRI neck for assessment of soft tissue
    - CT neck (may miss radiolucent calculi)
5. Management
    - Conservative: Hydration, gland massage, sialogogues
    - Medical: Antibiotics for acute infections, analgesia
    - Surgical:
        - Sialendoscopy: LA, sedation or GA, for stones <4 mm
        - Interventional: Contrast localisation, basket retrieval, duct dilatation/stent
        - Intra-oral retrieval:
            - ■ Suture behind calculus to prevent displacement
            - ■ Incision over calculus
            - ■ Evert and suture edges to prevent stenosis

- SMG excision:
  - For chronic, recurrent symptoms and failed conservative/medical management
  - Larger calculi
  - Intraglandular calculus

Grave's Disease

1. Background:
   - Grave's disease: Thyroid-stimulating immunoglobulins (TSIs) via TSH receptors. Raised T3 and T4
   - Thyroid eye disease: Lymphocytic infiltration in orbital fat and extra-ocular muscles increasing orbital volume
   - Thyroid storm:
     - Life-threatening hypermetabolic state, with 90% mortality. Can be first presentation of hyperthyroidism
     - Related to stress (sepsis, surgery, infection)
     - Pyrexia >40, tachycardia (arrhythmia), hypertension, eventual CCF, anxiety, GI disturbances (diarrhoea), coma
2. History:
   - Related to hypermetabolic state:
     - General: Fatigue, irritability, thin hair, hyperhidrosis, heat intolerance, weight loss
     - Cardiology: Tachycardia, arrhythmias
     - Respiratory: Dyspnoea (CCF or arrhythmia)
     - Neurology: Coarse tremor, proximal weakness
     - GI: Diarrhoea
     - Psychiatry: Anxiety/depression
   - Eye symptoms: Lid lag, lid retraction, proptosis/exophthalmos, ophthalmoplegia
   - Compressive symptoms: SOB, stridor, dysphagia
   - Radiation exposure
3. Examination:
   - Head and neck: Assess for goitre
   - Ophthalmology: Assess for thyroid eye signs (as above)
   - Hands and systemic
4. Investigations:
   - TFT's, TSI (anti-TSH, anti-TPO, anti-Tg)
   - USS neck ± FNAC: High risk for differentiated thyroid cancer
   - Visual acuity: Ophthalmology referral

5. Management:
   - Medical:
     - MDT approach (endocrine, ophthalmology)
     - Treatment with radioactive iodine (I-131) focuses on metabolically active regions within thyroid
       - Contraindicated in pregnancy
       - Risk of hypothyroidism: Destroys thyroid tissue
       - Not to breastfeed until next pregnancy
       - Not to conceive for 6 months
     - Carbimazole or propylthiouracil (faster) inhibits iodination/organification of Tyrosine, required to synthesis T3 and T4, reduces T4 release. Duration 12–18 months. During pregnancy, PTU for first trimester
       - Agranulocytosis occurs in <1% of case
       - Other SE's: Fever, rash, arthralgia, GI disturbance, alopecia, loss of taste and hepatic disturbance
       - If Carbimazole is contraindicated, lithium (inhibits TH secretion and Iodine coupling) – monitoring required
     - Steroids for thyroid eye disease as initial management
   - Surgical:
     - MDT approach (endocrine, surgeon, anaesthetist)
     - Beta blockade 6–8 weeks prior to surgery (40 mg TDS-QDS)
     - Render euthyroid several weeks prior to operation
     - Lugol's pre-op: 10 days
     - Total thyroidectomy
       - Indications:
         - Compressive symptoms
         - Refractory to medical treatment (50% relapse) or toxicity from medical treatment or storm
         - Not candidate for radioiodine therapy (pregnancy)
         - Thyroid eye disease: Reduction in antithyroid antibodies/fibroblast activity
         - Suspected malignancy on USS/FNAC
       - Complications:
         - Pain, infection, bleeding, haematoma, scarring, hypocalcaemia (10% transient), hypothyroidism (1%), recurrence, RLN injury (1%), unilateral or bilateral, necessitating tracheostomy
     - Thyroid eye disease:
       - Surgical decompression: Medial orbital decompression (endoscopic), infero-medial strut to prevent diplopia

Treatment of thyroid storm

- MDT approach: Endocrinology, cardiology, ITU, surgical (life-threatening emergency):
- Conservative:
  - Cooling blankets
- Medical:
  - ITU admission
  - Fluids (Dextrose due to metabolic demands) and electrolyte correction
  - Carbimazole/PTU (as per Grave's)
  - Lugol's
  - Propranolol (Metoprolol): Prevents conversion of T4 to T3
  - Steroids (adrenal exhaustion)
  - Iodine or lithium: Reduce and inhibit thyroid release (Wolff-Chaikoff effect)
- Surgical:
  - Total thyroidectomy once patient has been medically stabilised

Post-operative Hypocalcaemia

1. Background:
   - Normal range 2.20–2.60 mmol/l
   - Daily Ca intake – 1g (max 2g)
   - Mainly transient (10%) but can be permanent
   - Aim to keep within range 2.00–2.30
   - Can be associated with hyperphosphataemia and hypomagnesaemia
   - Vitamin D synthesis:
     - In skin:
       - 7-Dehydrocholesterol + UV = Cholecalciferol (pre-vitamin D3)
     - In liver:
       - 25 Hydroxylase + Cholecalciferol = 25-hydroxycholecalciferol (25-hydroxyvitamin D3) = calcidiol
     - In kidney:
       - 25-hydroxycholecalciferol + 1-alpha-hydroxylase = 1,25-dihydroxycholecalciferol (1,25-dihydroxyvitamin D3) = calcitriol
       - Alfacalcidol (Calcichew-D3 is with addition of Ca) = 1-alpha-hydroxycholecalciferol = analogue of vitamin D, but weaker
         - It is an active metabolite, hence a second hydroxylation is not required
         - Commonly given to end-stage renal disease patients as are unable to hydroxylate

        - Effects: Increases serum Ca
            - Small bowel and renal re-absorption of Ca (at collecting ducts and distal tubules)
            - Release of Ca from bone
    - Function of PTH:
        - Secreted by chief cells of parathyroid gland
        - Reduces serum phosphate through reduced renal re-absorption
        - Increases serum calcium through action on:
            - Bone: Through direct activation of osteoclasts
            - Renal: Up-regulates 1-alpha-hydroxylation of 25-hydroxyvitamin D3 to 1,25-Dihydroxyvitamin D3
            - GI tract: Increased absorption of Ca from gut via 1,25-Dihydroxyvitamin D3

2. History:
    - Circumoral tingling
    - Peripheral tingling/paraesthesia
    - SOB, indicative of arrhythmia
    - Stridor indicative of laryngospasm
    - Tetany/spasm
3. Examination:
    - Evidence of neuromuscular irritability:
        - Chvostek's (tapping on facial nerve elicits facial twitching)
        - Trousseau's (carpopedal spasm following blood pressure cuff inflation)
4. Investigations:
    - Serum calcium and PTH, phosphate
    - Magnesium, as can be associated with hypocalcaemia
    - ECG: Prolonged QT interval
5. Management:
    - BAETS guidance:
        - Treat all patients who are symptomatic, with method dependent on levels of calcium and severity of symptoms
            - 2.01–2.10 mmol/l: Observe, and re-check in 24 hrs
            - 1.81–2.00 mmol/l: Initiate oral therapy in a stepwise manner:
Sandocal = 1 g calcium (Ca^2+ 25 mmol)
Alfacalcidol = 1–2 mcg in divided doses or OD
Calcium and alfacalcidol: Calcichew D3 (1 tab TDS)
            - ≤1.80 mmol/l: IV calcium as below
    - Treat any patient with symptoms or calcium <1.80, even if asymptomatic
        - ECG – HDU with cardiac monitoring
        - 10 mL 10% Ca gluconate in 100 mL saline over 1 hrs
        - 40 mL 10% Ca gluconate in 1000 mL saline over 24 hrs

    - Oral calcium once in range
  - Treatment either with calcium, or addition of alfacalcidol (1–2 mcg OD or in divided dose)

Hypercalcaemia (Hyperparathyroidism)

1. Background:
   - Parafollicular cells (C cells) of thyroid: Reduce osteoclastic activity and renal re-absorption of Ca, hence reducing serum calcium
   - Chief cells of PT glands; increase osteoclastic activity and renal re-absorption of Ca, as well as hydroxylation of 25-Vit-D3, raising serum calcium
   - Normal range: 2.20–2.60
   - Defined as serum Ca > 2.60 on two occasions:
     - Mild: 2.60–3.00
     - Moderate: 3.01–3.40
     - Severe: 3.40 (urgent treatment required)
   - Due to excess PTH, secondary to parathyroid adenoma (single in 80% of cases) or multi-gland hyperplasia (19% due to MEN 1 and 2a, and familial hypocalciuric hypercalcaemia), tertiary hyperparathyroidism, parathyroid cancer, other rare causes (i.e. ectopic ACTH secreting lung source, Cushing's syndrome)
   - Indications for excision:
     - Ca >2.85
     - Symptomatic
     - eGFR <60
     - Resistant to medical therapy
     - Osteoporosis
2. History:
   - Most patients are asymptomatic, but usually:
     - Renal stones
     - Polyuria and polydipsia
     - Joint and muscle pain
     - Constipation, ulcers
     - Depression/fatigue
     - Fractures
3. Examination:
   - Cognitive impairment
   - Full head and neck examination
4. Investigations:
   - Serum calcium, PTH, Mg as a baseline
   - Baseline ECG, for reduced QT interval

- Mainly diagnosed on radiological correlation, which is a combination of two scans:
  - USS
  - Radiolabelled Tc-99m sestamibi scan (when combined with USS neck, has a sensitivity of 95%)
  - SPECT (usually different acquisition camera when compared to sestamibi, but adds CT for better anatomy. 2–3% higher accuracy compared to sestamibi)
  - 2 hrs post-washout phase: Out of thyroid but remains in parathyroid adenoma (high mitochondrial concentration)
  - 4D-CT, with fourth dimension being time. 50× radiation dose
  - MRI rarely
  - If still inconclusive then 4 gland exploration

5. Management:
   - Surgical resection is definitive (Risk: Hungry bone syndrome – rebound hypocalcaemia)
     - Adenoma excision
     - Subtotal resection for hyperplasia
     - 4 gland exploration where imaging discordant
       - ■ Confirmation with:
         - o Frozen section
         - o Intra-operative PTH (three levels): Pre-induction, pre-excision, 20 min post-excision. Confirmation of successful resection if >50% drop in PTH levels and within normal limit
         - o Remove all four glands if cannot localise
   - Medical management:
     - IV rehydration (0.9% Saline, 4–6 l/24 hrs)
     - Bisphosphonates (Pamidronate 30–90 mg)
     - Calcitonin
     - Cinacalcet (activates Ca receptors on PT gland to produce negative feedback)
     - Loop diuretics (furosemide)
     - Steroids (inhibits 1, 25OH vitamin D production, reduce intestinal absorption, 40 mg prednisolone)
     - Haemodialysis for advanced or life-threatening disease

Multiple Endocrine Neoplasia

1. Background:
   - MEN is a group of disorders affecting hormone-producing glands characterised by patterns of benign and malignant growths (Table 1.4)
   - Grouped as MEN1, MEN2A and MEN2B

Table 1.4 Multiple Endocrine Neoplasia Findings

MEN 1 (Werner's Syndrome)	*MEN 2A (Sipple Syndrome) (1M 2Ps)*	*MEN 2B 2Ms 1P*
Parathyroid hyperplasia: Most common presentation (95%, mainly under 30 years of age) Pituitary adenomas: prolactinoma, TSH-oma, non-functioning Pancreatic tumours: VIP-oma, insulinoma, gastrinoma, non-functioning)	Medullary thyroid cancer (thyroidectomy aged 6 years of age) Parathyroid hyperplasia Phaeochromocytoma	Medullary thyroid cancer (thyroidectomy in infancy >90% risk) Marfanoid habitus Mucosal neuromas Phaeochromocytoma

   - MEN1 have MEN mutations
   - MEN2A and MEN2B have RET mutations, with MEN2B associated with more aggressive medullary thyroid disease
2. History:
   - MEN syndrome patients can present to ENT with symptoms of thyroid gland enlargement (medullary thyroid cancer) or hypercalcaemia from parathyroid hyperplasia
   - They can also be identified through family genetic screening
   - Hyperparathyroidism is the normal presentation for MEN1
   - Medullary thyroid cancer (or phaeochromocytoma) is the normal presentation for MEN2
3. Examination:
   - Thyroid and H&N examination
4. Investigations:
   - Serum calcium and PTH
   - Calcitonin and CEA levels (pre-operatively)
   - Plasma-free normetanephrine
   - USS FNAC for thyroid nodules
   - CT or MRI for staging medullary thyroid cancer
   - RET proto-oncogene analysis (post-operatively)
5. Management:
   - Management should be governed by an MDT experienced in the management of neuroendocrine tumours
   - Medullary thyroid cancer:
     - Patients with medullary thyroid cancer >5 mm should have a total thyroidectomy and central compartment neck dissection

    - With lateral nodal disease, or central node mets, patients should undergo selective neck dissection (IIa–V)
    - Genetic counselling and testing
  - Family genetic screening for RET oncogene
    - Prophylactic thyroidectomy for RET-positive family members
    - Generally, for MEN2A should be arranged <5 years old and for MEN2B <1 years old
  - Pre-operative medical management of phaeochromocytoma
  - Surgical management of parathyroid disease: Usually multiple/four-gland disease
  - For MEN1, fasting GI tract hormone blood tests, including gastrin, glucagon, vasointestinal polypeptide, pancreatic polypeptide, chromogranin A, insulin and glucose
6. Differential diagnoses:
  - Non-syndromic disease

Thyroid Cancer

1. Background:
  - Well-differentiated thyroid cancer:
    - Papillary thyroid carcinoma:
      - 80% of thyroid malignancies
      - Associated with previous radiation
      - Spread to lymphatics
      - <1 cm is a papillary microcarcinoma: Adequately treated with hemithyroidectomy alone
    - Follicular thyroid carcinoma:
      - Second most common thyroid cancer
      - Haematogenous spread (rare to lymph nodes)
      - Differentiation of carcinoma from adenoma depends on capsular invasion
    - Hurtle cell carcinoma:
      - Previously considered a variant of follicular carcinoma, now a category in its own right
      - Worse prognosis than follicular thyroid cancer
    - Anaplastic thyroid cancer:
      - Undifferentiated thyroid cancer
      - Likely dedifferentiation from papillary or follicular thyroid cancer
      - Affects the elderly, rapidly progressing
      - Very poor prognosis, can compromise airway
      - Surgical intervention generally not indicated (not curative) as disease often very advanced

- Medullary thyroid cancer:
  - ■ Originates from the parafollicular (C) cells
  - ■ 75% sporadic, 25% genetic (autosomal dominant)
    - o MEN 2A and 2B syndrome and familial medullary thyroid carcinoma
    - o RET mutation
  - ■ Pre-operatively needs calcitonin and carcinoembryonic antigen (CEA)
    - o Pentagastrin-stimulated calcitonin if calcitonin mildly elevated
  - ■ Once medullary thyroid cancer diagnosed needs pre-operatively:
    - o Plasma normetanephrines (exclude phaeochromocytoma)
    - o Serum calcium (exclude hyperparathyroidism)
  - ■ Post-operatively needs RET gene mutation sequencing
    - o Genetic counselling and consideration of family screening
  - ■ Common lymphatic and distant metastatic spread
- Lymphoma
  - ■ Diagnosed on core biopsy or open biopsy

2. History:
   - Onset, progression of symptoms
   - Swallowing or airway issues
   - Voice change
   - PMH:
     - Autoimmune thyroid disease, previous radiation exposure
     - Family history thyroid cancer
3. Examination:
   - Head and neck examination: Size of thyroid/nodule, movement with swallowing, retrosternal extension, neck nodes
   - Flexible nasolaryngoscopy: VC function
4. Investigations:
   - Thyroid function tests and autoantibodies
   - Calcitonin and CEA in medullary thyroid cancer
   - USS ± FNAC (based on size and U classification on ultrasound – Figure 1.3)
     - Features of malignancy: Solid, hypo-echoic, irregular outline, micro-calcification, metastatic nodes
   - CT neck and chest if considered to be retrosternal
   - CT or MRI neck for staging if clinical nodes apparent or if medullary
5. Management:
   - All thyroid cancers should be managed within an MDT setting
   - Differentiated thyroid cancer (papillary and follicular thyroid carcinoma) is initially managed based on the outcomes from USS and FNAC (Table 1.5)

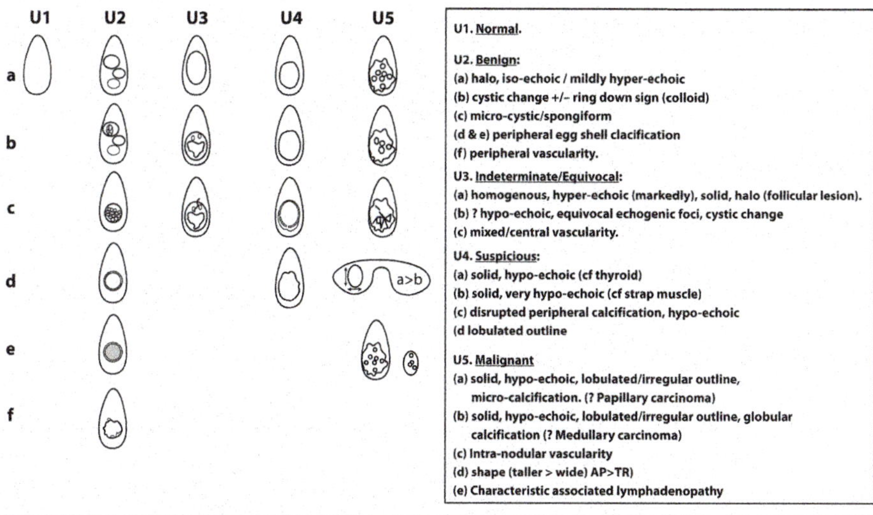

Figure 1.3 Ultrasound characteristics of thyroid lesions.

Table 1.5 The Cytological Classification for Differentiated Thyroid Cancer

Thy Category	*Description*	*% Malignancy*	*Management*
Thy1 **Thy1c**	Non-diagnostic for cytological diagnosis Non-diagnostic for cytological diagnosis – cystic lesion	0–10	Repeat FNAC
Thy2 **Thy2c**	Non-neoplastic Non-neoplastic – cystic lesion	0–3	Review clinical and US level of suspicion
Thy3a **Thy3f**	Neoplasm possible. – atypia/ non-diagnostic Neoplasm possible, suggesting follicular neoplasm	5–15 15–30	Further investigation – USS ± repeat FNAC Diagnostic hemithyroidectomy
Thy4	Suspicious of malignancy	60–75	Diagnostic hemithyroidectomy
Thy5	Malignant	97–100	Therapeutic thyroidectomy

Table 1.6 Prognostic Risk Score for Differentiated Thyroid Cancer

Ages	*Ames*	*MACIS: Low Risk if <6 (Deemed Cured)*
Age Grade Extent of disease Size	Age Metastasis Extent of disease Size	Metastasis: Yes (3), no (0) Age: <39 (3.1), >40 (0.08 × age) Completeness of excision: Complete (0), incomplete (1) Invasion (surrounding tissue): Yes (1), no (0) Size: 0.3 × size (cm)

- Those who have a hemithyroidectomy which diagnoses a differentiated carcinoma may need completion thyroidectomy and central neck dissection (not needed if unifocal, contained to thyroid, <4 cm, negative nodes and low risk): this facilitates post-operative ablative therapy with radioactive iodine. Prognostic risk factors are taken into consideration for personalised decision making on treatment (Table 1.6)
- Lateral neck dissection is only indicated in the presence of disease – level IIa–Vb, preserving SCM, IJV and accessory nerve
- Immediately, post-operatively all total or completion thyroidectomy patients need calcium/PTH checks and thyroxine replacement (2 mcg/kg)
- Post-operative radioactive iodine:
  - Indications: >4 cm, vascular invasion, extrathyroidal spread or metastasis
  - Side effects: Dry eyes/mouth, fatigue, nausea, sialadenitis (long term: infertility, secondary cancers)
  - During treatment: Avoid direct contact with children for 2 weeks, women not to conceive a pregnancy for 6 months, stop breastfeeding, men not to father children for 4 months
- Post-operatively dynamic risk stratification is undertaken 9 months after surgery for patients who have had total thyroidectomy and RAI
  - Stimulated thyroglobulin and ultrasound scan (± radioactive iodine scan)
  - Excellent/indeterminate/incomplete response which correlates with low/intermediate/high risk (Table 1.7)
  - Determines whether TSH suppression with thyroxine is required

– Medullary thyroid cancer:
  - Pre-operative investigations as above
  - Total thyroidectomy and central compartment neck dissection (levels VI and VII)
    - Ipsilateral prophylactic lateral neck dissection if central compartment node positive (risk of nodal disease 70%)

Table 1.7 Post-Treatment Dynamic Risk Stratification from British Thyroid Association 2014 Guidelines

Excellent Response	*Indeterminate Response*	*Incomplete Response*
All the following • Suppressed and stimulated Tg < 1 lg/l* • Neck US without evidence of disease • Cross-sectional and/or nuclear medicine imaging negative (if performed)	Any of the following • Suppressed Tg < 1 lg/l and stimulated Tg ≥1 and <10 lg/l • Neck US with non-specific changes or stable sub-centimetre lymph nodes • Cross-sectional and/or nuclear medicine imaging with non-specific changes, although not completely normal	Any of the following • Suppressed Tg≥1 lg/l* or stimulated Tg ≥ 10 lg/l* • Rising Tg values • Persistent or newly identified disease on cross-sectional and/or nuclear medicine imaging
TSH to be maintained in low-normal range 0.3–2 mU/l	TSH suppression to 0.1–0.5 mU/l for 5–10 years and then reassess	TSH suppressed below 0.1 mU/l indefinitely

Note: *Assumes the absence of interference in the Tg assay.

    - Personalised decision-making regarding prophylactic bilateral neck dissections (improves post-operative calcitonin, impact on survival unknown)
    - Even those with distant metastasis should have local surgery to prevent invasion of local structures as often prolonged survival
  - Family genetic counselling if genetic:
    - Children with MEN2B should have prophylactic thyroidectomy within first year of life
    - Children with MEN2A should have prophylactic thyroidectomy before 5 years
- Anaplastic thyroid cancer:
  - Best results are from surgical resection plus radical external beam radiation and chemotherapy
  - Majority will not have disease amenable to radical treatment
  - Survival is 3–7 months
  - Benefits of any interventions should be discussed at MDT
  - Consider for clinical trials: Combination of targeted therapies is under investigation
  - Palliative care referral as indicated

6. Differential diagnoses:
   - Thyroglossal duct cyst (differentiated by movement on tongue protrusion and USS)
7. Evidence:
   - HiLo trial: Dehbi et al. Recurrence after low-dose radioiodine ablation and recombinant human thyroid-stimulating hormone for differentiated thyroid cancer (HiLo): Long-term results of an open-label, non-inferiority randomised controlled trial. Lancet 2018; 7(1): 44–51
     - No significant increase in recurrence between low-dose 1.1 vs 3.7 GBq radioiodine administration

Assessment of Parotid Mass

1. Background:
   - 80% of salivary tumours are parotid in origin
   - 80% of parotid, 70% of submandibular and 50% of sublingual tumours and 30% minor salivary gland tumours are benign
   - 80% pleomorphic adenoma
2. History:
   - Timing (onset and periodicity)
   - Size (increase or fluctuance)
   - Association with meals
   - Other masses (metastatic disease)
   - Systemic features (inflammatory origin or lymphoproliferative disorder), dysphagia, dysphonia, odynophagia or dyspnoea
   - Associated pain or facial weakness (malignancy), bleeding, trismus
   - PMH:
     - Previous head and neck surgery/treatment (radiotherapy-induced malignancy or recurrence)
     - Previous skin malignancy, especially SCC
   - SH: Smoking and drinking
3. Examination:
   - Full head and neck examination, focusing on mass to assess for mobility, fixation, contour and presence of a smaller mass on the opposite side (Warthin's tumour)
   - Tonsil medialisation
   - Examination of scalp
   - Facial nerve
4. Investigations:
   - USS + FNAC/core biopsy
   - MRI neck: Fat suppressed STIR sequence to determine deep lobe involvement
   - CT thorax to exclude distant metastasis

5. Management:
   - Medical (limited role):
     - If malignant and unfit for surgery then option for primary RT
     - Post-operative RT for high-grade cancer features (see Table 1.8)
     - May need no intervention if Warthin's tumour
   - Surgical:
     - Risks: GA, pain, infection, bleeding, scarring, numbness, facial weakness (20% temporary, 1% permanent), sialocoele, salivary fistula, gustatory sweating (treat with antiperspirant/Botox/TF graft/Jacobson neurectomy), first bite syndrome, cosmetic deformity

Table 1.8 Salivary Gland Neoplasia Differential Diagnosis and Management

Benign	*Malignant*
Pleomorphic adenoma: Females > males Most common parotid and lacrimal gland tumour Malignancy: 1% per year cumulative up to 10% over 15 years Management: Superficial parotidectomy (if in superficial lobe)	**Mucoepidermoid tumour:** Most common malignant major salivary gland tumour with >90% in parotid Most common malignant salivary gland tumour (low grade) in children Histologically divided into low, intermediate and high grade which correlates with prognosis 5-yr survival 86% low grade and 22% high grade Management: Surgical excision Elective neck dissection indicated for high-grade tumours Post-operative radiotherapy for residual disease or if > 4 cm
Warthin's tumour (papillary cystadenoma lymphomatosum): Middle-aged men, elderly Smoking association and alcohol association 10% bilateral Rare outside parotid PET positive due to high mitochondrial concentration Management: Observation alone or superficial parotidectomy (if in superficial lobe)	**Adenoid cystic carcinoma:** Three histological growth patterns: Tubular, cribriform and solid (solid worst prognosis) Common in submandibular gland/minor salivary glands Slow onset, peri-neural invasion – associated with CN VII palsy and neuralgic pain Nodal spread rare (4%) Distant metastasis (lungs) frequently occur, and can be late (after 5-yrs disease-free) <20% 5-yr survival in high-grade tumours Management: Wide local excision with preservation of uninvolved nerves Post-operative radiotherapy

(Continued)

Table 1.8 Salivary Gland Neoplasia Differential Diagnosis and Management *(Continued)*

Benign	*Malignant*
Oncocytoma: Rare benign tumour of mitochondria-rich oncocytes 1% of salivary gland neoplasms Rare outside parotid	**Acinic cell carcinoma:** Parotid mainly Can be bilateral in 3% 80% are low grade with 90% 5-yr survival Management: Total parotidectomy preservation of uninvolved nerves (no elective neck dissection, radiotherapy can be considered)
	Lymphoma: Rare as primary site, arising from intraglandular lymphoid tissue NH lymphoma association
	SCC: Rare as a primary site, evaluate as for metastasis from primary skin SCC Management: Radical resection with adjuvant radiotherapy
	Carcinoma ex-pleomorphic adenoma (malignant mixed tumour): Broad category of carcinomas of salivary ducts Only a minority arise from pleomorphic adenoma High recurrence rate Categorised as in situ, non-invasive, minimally invasive (<1.5 mm) and invasive
	Salivary duct carcinoma: Rare, accounting for 2% of all salivary gland malignancies HER2 positive 15-40%, Androgen receptor positive 67-97% Highly aggressive with poor prognosis Management: wide surgical excision, neck dissection and adjuvant radiotherapy. Targeted immunotherapy should be considered based on the molecular characteristics of the tumour.
Management summary: Manage malignant tumours within the head and neck MDT N+ necks should have a neck dissection (based on stage and location), N0 neck if high grade, >4 cm or SCC Post-operative radiotherapy for tumours which are high grade, >4 cm, positive margins, extracapsular spread, after surgery for recurrent disease and for adenoid cystic carcinoma	

6. Differential diagnoses:
   - Inflammatory:
     - Parotitis/sialadenitis, usually 60% due to sialolithiasis. Organism usually *S. aureus*. Triggered by dehydration. Medically managed
     - Mumps: Paramyxovirus. May be unilateral. Conservative management
   - Systemic:
     - Sjogren's syndrome (unilateral or bilateral). Lymphocytic infiltration of exocrine glands
     - Sarcoidosis: Heerfordt syndrome (Uveoparotid fever, associated with facial nerve palsy and uveitis)
     - HIV: Lymphoepithelial cysts. Conservatively managed
   - Neoplastic (see Table 1.8)

Facial nerve landmarks:

- Approximately, 1 cm anterior, deep and inferior to tragal pointer (variable soft tissue landmark)
- 6–8 mm deep to the lateral aspect of the tympanomastoid suture line
- Posterior belly of digastric at same depth as facial nerve, anteromedial to it at mastoid insertion
- Mastoid exploration
- Retrograde identification:
  - MMN
  - Zygomatic branch crosses midpoint of arch
  - Buccal 1 cm parallel and inferior to Stenson's duct

Facial nerve monitor: 0.25–0.5mA

Oral Malignancy

1. Background:
   - Nodal spread levels I–III
   - Most common malignancy of the H&N
     - Tongue: Most common oral cavity cancer in the UK
     - Lower lip bilateral lymphatic drainage into levels I–III, hence high stage requires bilateral neck treatment
     - Upper lip ipsilateral into levels I–III (poorer prognosis, closer to critical structures adjacent to nasal cavity)
   - Floor of mouth second most common in the UK, followed be alveolar margin, buccal and lip (2-3%). Worldwide lip is recorded as most common followed by oral tongue.
   - Usually exophytic mass

- Rule of 90s:
    - 90% SCC (non-SCC: Melanoma, sarcoma, salivary gland), 90% lower lip and 90% 5-yr survival if T1
    - BCC upper lip (closer to UV exposure), common in females
- Other cancers: Minor salivary (mucoepidermoid, adenoid cystic, adenocarcinoma)
- Up to 20% of early stage oral cancers harbour occult nodal metastasis, hence need for treatment to neck. Overall 30%. Sites with <20% occult metastatic rate to the neck are: T1/2 lip, T1/2 oral tongue and <4mm thick, T1/2 floor of mouth and ≤ 1.5mm thick.

T category	Features
Tis	Carcinoma in situ
T1	Tumour ≤2 cm
T2	Tumour >2cm but ≤4cm
T3	Tumour >4 cm
T4a	Tumour invades the larynx, deep/extrinsic muscles of tongue, medial pterygoid (closer to primary), hard palate or mandible
T4b	Tumour invades lateral pterygoid (further distance), pterygoid plates, lateral nasopharynx or skull base or encases carotid

2. History:
    - Non-healing ulcers (>2 weeks), dysphagia, odynophagia, referred otalgia, trismus (pterygoid involvement), lower teeth numbness (inferior alveolar nerve involvement), bleeding, loose teeth, neck lumps
    - PMH: Dental hygiene, past history of leukoplakia, erythroplakia, previous malignancy/treatment of head and neck, trauma
    - SH: 5 S's: Smoking, spirits, spices (betel nut), syphilis, sharp tooth (chronic inflammation)
3. Examination:
    - Full head and neck examination, assessing oropharyngeal lesion (lateral, crossing midline)
        - Assessment for trismus, which would indicate advanced disease
        - Assessment for regional/nodal involvement
        - Flexible nasolaryngoscopy for second primary
4. Investigations:
    - OPG: Mental foramen positioning and height of mandible (rim resection)
    - Advanced: MRI (soft tissue delineation)/CT for staging purposes (neck and chest) as well as bony involvement
    - Sentinel node biopsy for early stage oral cancers, may negate need for ND (if early stage/small T1 tumours)

5. Management:
   - All treatments should be discussed at local MDT
   - Surgery is primary modality of choice, with 1cm clearance required, CRT only in advanced disease due to associated morbidity (osteoradionecrosis) and severe mucositis with oral fibrosis
   - <5-mm margin: Discuss at MDT? re-excision or RT
   - Anterior tumours accessed transorally, posterior tumours with tongue release or lip split mandibulotomy
   - Treatment to neck is required if occult metastatic risk is >20% (most oral cancers, except some T1 <3-mm depth of invasion). Level 1 evidence of improved survival with elective neck dissection in N0 disease
   - Treatment to neck not usually performed in lip cancers (5% risk of occult metastasis) unless clinically evident nodes (poor prognostic factor)
   - Reconstruction:
     - Small lesions: Partial glossectomy and primary closure/secondary intention if <30% tongue volume loss
     - Pedicled: Submental island flap (submental artery from facial), nasolabial flap or pec major for large defect
     - Large defects: Total glossectomy + free flaps: Radial forearm or ALT
     - Osseocutaneous: Scapular, fibula flap
     - Oral:
       - T1–T2: Resection + SND (I–III ±IV) or very rarely brachytherapy (small primary) or EBRT
       - T3–T4 (N1): Resection + neck dissection (reconstruction) + PORT ± concurrent chemotherapy (ECS/+ve margins)
         - Bilateral neck if crossing or 1 cm from midline. MRND if multiple nodes, bulky disease or ECS
         - Abutment of mandible may require marginal mandibulectomy, involvement requires segmental resection
         - Marginal mandibulectomy: RFFF reconstruction
         - Segmental resection: Lip split incision for access. Fibula or scapula free flap for reconstruction.
     - Lip:
       - T1–T4 Resection or RT/brachytherapy
       - For early stages: Surgery and RT, same outcomes. Surgery is mainstay of treatment. 5-mm margins
       - Resections:
         - Upper lip:
           - <1/2: Wedge resection and primary closure
           - 1/2–2/3: Perialar crescentic flap (advancement flap)
Reverse Karapandzic flap
Bilateral Gillies fan flap (nasolabial transposition flap)

- o Lower lip:
  - – <1/2: Wedge resection and primary closure
  - – 1/2–2/3: Peri-alar crescentic flap (advancement flap)
  - – 1/2–2/3: Karapandzic
    Bernard-Burrow

Oropharyngeal Malignancy

1. Background:
   - 95% SCC, lymphoma
   - Tonsil most common. Tongue base: HPV most common cause. Poorer prognosis and more aggressive if HPV negative
     - Double-stranded DNA virus, which infects stratified squamous epithelium. Type 16 most common
     - L1 (capsid protein of HPV) and L2 are proteins that encapsulate viral particle
     - E6 and E7 are proto-oncogenes responsible for anogenital and H&N cancers
       - ■ E6 protein binds to and inactivates p53 tumour suppressor protein
       - ■ E7 protein binds to and inactivates Rb protein. Degradation of Rb protein is linked to p16 overexpression, which is used as a surrogate marker of HPV related SCC.
     - Not all p16 +ve results means HPV infection (10–20% not HPV +ve), p16 positivity in >70% of cells for confirmation
     - Improved overall survival and decreased loco-regional failure. Younger patients and non-smokers
     - Staging adjusted to downgrade overall stage to reflect improved survival despite more advanced disease with wider lymphadenopathy spread
     - Prognosis: HPV + non-smoker > HPV + smoker, HPV– and non-smoker > HPV– and smoker

Non-HPV oropharyngeal (OPC) staging: Addition on TNM 8

T category	Features
T1	Tumour <=2 cm, one subsite
T2	Tumour >2 cm <=4 cm, more than one subsite
T3	Tumour >4 cm
T4a	Extrinsic muscles of tongue, larynx or extension to lingual surface of epiglottis, hard palate, mandible
T4b	Involvement of lateral pterygoid plates, skull base, encasing carotid

N category	Features
N1	Single ipsilateral node <3 cm
N2a	Single ipsilateral node >3 cm but ≤6 cm
N2b	Multiple ipsilateral nodes >3 cm but ≤6 cm
N2c	Bilateral or contralateral nodes >3 cm but ≤6 cm
N3a	Metastasis in node >6 cm, without extra-nodal extension (ENE)
N3b	Metastasis in node >6 cm, with extra-nodal extension (ENE)

HPV + OPV:

N category	Features
Nx/0	Unable to assess/no regional nodes
N1	One ipsilateral node <=6 cm
N2	Contralateral or bilateral nodes <=6 cm
N3	Nodes >6 cm

2. History:
   - Presenting complaint:
     - Weight loss/nutritional status, fevers
     - Red flag symptoms: Dysphagia, dysphonia, dyspnoea, odynophagia, trismus, referred otalgia, globus, neck mass
   - Past medical history:
     - Previous head and neck cancer and treatment
   - Social history:
     - Smoking/drinking
     - Wider social support
3. Examination:
   - Full head and neck examination, assessing oropharyngeal lesion (lateral, crossing midline), nodal disease, trismus and extent with nasolaryngoscopy
   - Palpate tonsil and tongue base
   - Ear examination
4. Investigations:
   - USS neck + core biopsy
   - Cross-sectional imaging:
     - CT neck and thorax
     - MRI of primary for evaluation and treatment planning
     - Histological evaluation (panendoscopy + biopsy)
     - PET-CT for treatment response at 3–4/12 for advanced disease N2/3
5. Management:
   - MDT: Radiology/oncology/SALT/dietician/CNS
   - Conservative: Patient's wishes or not fit
   - Medical: RT mainstay for oropharynx (IMRT)

- HPV+: Where surgery as a unimodality treatment is possible, TORS or TLM with neck dissection is offered. Multimodality treatment is best delivered within clinical trials. Hence, TORS favoured for small lesions.
- De-escalate trials: No evidence to support de-escalation of treatment in an attempt to reduce toxicity
  - RT + cetuximab worse outcomes than RT+ cisplatin in HPV+
- PATHOS trial: Still in phase III – reducing RT dose post TORS in HPV+ T1–T3 oropharyngeal tumours to improve swallow function
- Early disease (T1–T2, N0): Single modality treatment recommended to primary and ipsilateral neck
  - T1–T2: Resection + SND (II-IV) OR IMRT to primary and neck (II–IV)
    - Excision via TORS or TLM method preferred due to better functional outcomes with a minimally invasive approach
    - Level II–IV ND and ligate lingual/facial artery. Then TORS to primary. Reduced severe bleeding rate
    - Post-operative (C)RT if adverse features
    - Always treat ipsilateral neck (10–30% occult)
    - Bilateral necks only if close to midline
- Advanced disease: Multi-modality treatment
  - T3–T4 (N1): Concurrent CRT or Resection (SND II-IV) + CRT
    - CRT mainstay of treatment but also consider trial recruitment if suitable surgical trials are open.
    - CRT if evidence of ECS, otherwise RT alone
    - Neck is treated even if N0 (surgery or RT)
    - Salvage procedure if CRT as first line fails
    - ND within 4 weeks if residual disease on post-treatment PET-CT; unequivocal PETCT findings can be observed for a further 2 to 3 months with repeat imaging.

Soft palate lesions:

- Differential diagnosis:
  - Benign: Pleomorphic, lipoma, haemangioma
  - Malignant: Mucoepidermoid/adenoid cystic/acinic cell/SCC/lymphoma
  - Mucous retention cyst
  - PNS tumour: JNA, Thornwaldt cyst, nasopharyngeal cancer, Antrochoanal polyp
- Considerations:
  - Hard palate involvement
  - Incisional biopsy
- Management:
  - The mainstay of treatment is primary radiotherapy
  - Surgical resection and reconstruction can be also considered but result in significant peri-operative (need for tracheostomy, nasogastric tube) and post-operative morbidity (speech/swallowing problems)

Laryngeal Malignancy

1. Background:
   - Supraglottic SCC:
     - 30–40% of laryngeal malignancies, with infrahyoid epiglottis most common site
     - Cancer usually spreads superiorly or into pre-epiglottic space
     - High rate of LN metastasis

T category	Features
T1	Confined to one subsite of supraglottis
T2	>1 subsite or glottis, or outside supraglottis (vallecula, tongue base, medial wall of piriform fossa)
T3	VF fixation. Invades post-cricoid, pre/para epiglottic space, inner cortex of thyroid cartilage
T4a	Outer cortex of thyroid cartilage, tissues beyond larynx
T4b	Prevertebral space/carotid involvement

- Glottic SCC:
  - 95% SCC
  - Broyles tendon: Anterior attachment of vocalis to thyroid cartilage – route of spread
  - Low rate of LN metastasis

T category	Features
T1a/b	Glottis, 1 vocal fold/glottis, bilateral vocal folds
T2a/b	Supra or subglottic spread. Impaired VF mobility distinguishes between T2a and T2b
T3	VF fixation (cricoarytenoid, vocalis involvement). Paraglottic spread. Inner cortex of cartilage
T4a	Outer cortex of thyroid cartilage, tissues beyond larynx
T4b	Prevertebral space/carotid involvement

- Subglottic SCC:
  - Rare primary site with poor prognosis
  - Subglottic lymph node drainage: Pre- and para-tracheal, prethyroidal and deep cervical chain

T category	Features
T1	Confined to subglottis
T2	Involvement of vocal folds. Impaired mobility
T3	VF fixation. Limited to larynx
T4a	Outer cortex of thyroid cartilage, tissues beyond larynx
T4b	Prevertebral space/carotid involvement

Nodal staging as listed in HPV –ve oropharyngeal malignancy

2. History:
   - Presenting complaint: Red flag symptoms: Dysphonia, dysphagia, odynophagia (supraglottis), dyspnoea, referred otalgia, stridor, weight loss, fevers
   - Past medical history: Previous head and neck cancer and treatment
   - Social history:
     - Smoking/drinking
     - Wider social support (likely needing laryngectomy, with subsequent stoma management consideration)
3. Examination:
   - Head and neck examination
     - Assessment for regional/nodal involvement
     - Flexible nasolaryngoscopy
4. Investigations:
   - USS ± core biopsy if any evidence of nodal disease
   - Cross-sectional imaging:
     - CT neck and thorax (can consider MRI of primary), although not indicated for T1 lesions (early cancer too small to be detected on imaging). Consider if extent difficult to assess
     - CT neck not needed for T1 glottic SCC
     - CT thorax: 5–10% synchronous lung primary
     - Histological evaluation (panendoscopy + biopsy)
5. Management:
   - All treatment should be discussed at local/regional MDT: Involvement of dieticians/SLT early if reduced oral intake
   - Treatment: Is always dependent on patient's performance status and wishes
     - Supraglottis:
       - T1–T2 (N0): Single modality and avoid dual modality due to impaired functional outcomes
         - Radiotherapy or TLM with bilateral elective neck treatment
       - If node +ve, RT or concurrent CRT (for advanced nodal disease) or RT following surgery
       - T3: Laryngeal preservation (non-surgical)
         - Concurrent CRT is standard of care
       - T4:
         - Total laryngectomy + bilateral elective neck (RT or neck dissection)
         - Consider CRT in very specific circumstances

- Glottis:
  - T1a–T2a: Single modality. Low incidence of neck disease and low tumour volume, hence neck not treated
    - Radiotherapy or TLM or open partial surgery (vertical partial, supracricoid)
    - For anterior commissure: Radical RT
  - T2b–T3 (N0): Laryngeal preservation (non-surgical)
    - CRT
    - Can consider laryngectomy if poor laryngeal function already
  - T4a:
    - Total laryngectomy if invasion through cartilage or poor laryngeal function + bilateral elective neck (RT or neck dissection).
    - Consider adjuvant CRT for adverse features

- If N2/3 disease: PET-CT post-CRT. Otherwise CT neck/chest at 3 months
- Post-operative radiotherapy to:
  - T4 disease
  - N2–N3 nodal disease
- Chemoradiotherapy if:
  - Close or +ve margins
  - Extracapsular spread

6. Evidence:
   - NICE: TLM for T1a
     - Same 5 year outcome with RT – 95%
     - Less morbidity (swallow)
     - RT backup
     - Single treatment that can be repeated
     - Disadvantages: Not possible in difficult access, potentially poorer voice outcomes
   - See Pignon et al. CT added to locoregional treatment for HNSCC: Meta-analysis of updated individual data. MACH-NC collaborative group. Lancet 2000; 355(9208):949–955
     - Concurrent CT to RT improves survival by 4% if under 71 years old, with increased toxicity
     - No survival benefit if over 71 years old
     - A 2021 update to the original paper, confirmed benefit/superiority of the addition of concomitant CT for non-metastatic head and neck cancer (Lacas B et al. Meta-analysis of chemotherapy in head and neck cancer (MACH-NC): An update on 107 randomized trials and 19,805 patients, on behalf of MACH-NC Group. Radiother Oncol. 2021 March;156:281–293)

Cordectomy types:

Type I: Subepithelium/epithelium + superficial lamina propria
Type II: Subligamentous + vocal ligament
Type III: Transmuscular + vocal ligament + vocalis muscle
Type IV: Total cordectomy (above plus all muscle to perichondrium, from vocal process to anterior commissure)
Type V cordectomy:

a. Anterior to contralateral cord
b. Posterior to arytenoids
c. Up to ventricle
d. Down to subglottis (1 cm)

Dysplasia management:

- Biopsies to ascertain degree of dysplasia
- Mapping biopsies if diffuse. Map accurately
- Three types:
  - Mild: Basal layer
  - Moderate: Mid spinous to basal
  - Severe: Superficial to basal (entire depth)
- Will progress to malignancy as follows:
  - Mild: 11% (can monitor along with moderate, but consider risk reduction)
  - Mild/moderate:
    - Focal: Excise
    - Diffuse: Can observe
  - Severe/cis: 25% can transform to invasive cancer. Endoscopic revision. Consider radiotherapy for persistent/ recurrent disease
  - Mild/moderate disease if excised and low risk (no visible lesion and smoking ceased for 6/12), can consider discharge after 6/12 follow-up and safety netting

Hypopharyngeal Malignancy

1. Background:
   - Three subsites (in order of most common):
     - Piriform fossa (75%), posterior pharyngeal wall (20%), post-cricoid (5% and more common in females – Plummer-Vinson)
   - Anatomically from superior aspect of hyoid to inferior border of cricoid

- Risk factors:
    - Smoking/drinking/tobacco, Barrett's oesophagus, LPR, Plummer-Vinson syndrome
- Poor prognosis due to:
    - Later presentation (stage III or IV disease in 80% of cases)
    - High likelihood of bilateral nodal disease, multi-level involvement or extracapsular spread
    - Highest rates of metastasis
    - 60% skip lesions
- Average 5-yr survival: 30%, 60% for early disease (T1/2)

T category	**Features**
Tis	Carcinoma in situ
T1	Tumour <=2 cm, one subsite
T2	Tumour >2 cm but <=4 cm, more than one subsite
T3	Tumour >4 cm, fixed vocal cord, oesophageal involvement
T4a	Tumour invades: Thyroid, cricoid, hyoid involvement or thyroid gland spread
T4b	Tumour invades: Prevertebral fascia, encasing carotid, mediastinal involvement

2. History:
    - Presenting complaint:
        - Weight loss/nutritional status
        - 60% present with a neck mass
        - Red flag symptoms: Dysphagia, dysphonia, dyspnoea, odynophagia, referred otalgia
    - Past medical history:
        - Previous head and neck treatment
    - Social history:
        - Smoking/drinking
        - Wider social support (likely needing laryngectomy, with subsequent stoma management consideration)
3. Examination:
    - Full head and neck examination, assessing oropharyngeal lesion (lateral, crossing midline)
        - Assessment for trismus, which would indicate advanced disease
        - Assessment for regional/nodal involvement
        - Flexible nasolaryngoscopy
4. Investigations:
    - Cross-sectional imaging:
        - CT neck and thorax (can consider MRI of primary)

- Histological evaluation (panendoscopy + biopsy)
- PET-CT indications:
  - ■ Recurrent disease, where radical treatment is planned
  - ■ Advanced disease (T4 or N3) and hypopharyngeal SCC

5. Management:
   - All treatment should be discussed at local/regional MDT: Involvement of dieticians/SLT early if reduced oral intake
   - Treatment: Is always dependent on patient's performance status and wishes
   - Tumour bulk can be reduced with neo-adjuvant CT
   - CRT offers organ preservation but has high short-term complications
   - If compromised swallow, consider surgery, due to side effects of CRT
     - Early disease (T1–T2 – not involving cartilage, lateral wall/apex of piriform fossa, oesophagus or cord fixation):
       - ■ Radical RT (with salvage) or surgical resection
       - ■ Where possible, consider endoscopic resection-laser or robotic (well-localised lesions)
       - ■ 30–40% occult neck nodes so elective ND
     - Advanced disease (T3–T4a):
       - ■ Surgical resection + ND + RT
       - ■ Bulky tumours should have circumferential excision (submucosal skip lesions)
       - ■ Offer surgery if compromised larynx or swallowing issues
       - ■ Total laryngectomy or pharyngolaryngectomy
         - o 3.5 cm of pharyngeal mucosa, primary closure
         - o 1–3.5 cm, consider pedicled flap
         - o <1 cm, total reconstruction with tubed ALT or jejunal graft
         - o If upper oesophagus involved: Gastric pull up
         - o Margins: 1.5 cm superior, 2 cm lateral, 3 cm inferior
     - Neck disease:
       - ■ Elective treatment to bilateral necks (levels II–IV) in midline lesions, medial piriform fossa, post-pharyngeal wall or post-cricoid lesions or node positive disease

The Unknown Primary

1. Background:
   - USS guided core for confirmation of SCC
   - Usually N2 at presentation
   - Cystic lesion in level II is a hallmark of HPV related SCC. P16 +ve lesions suggests likelihood of oropharynx as site

- Staged as T0, not Tx
- Important to find primary to reduce radiation volume

2. History:
   - Presentation: Usually asymptomatic, but may have had dysphagia, dysphonia, dyspnoea, odynophagia or otalgia prior to presentation, preceding illness, nasal symptoms, hearing reduction, weight loss, fevers
   - Details regarding nodal mass: Fluctuance in size, or rapidly progressive. Length of time present, other lumps
   - PMH: Previous cancer treatment (evidence of recurrence or secondary malignancy from previous radiotherapy)
   - SH: Smoking and drinking
3. Examination:
   - Head and neck examination comprising:
     - Oropharynx, including intra-oral palpation (tonsil, tongue base)
     - Skin/scalp as potential site
     - Palpation: Features of node, bilateral involvement or thyroid pathology
     - Flexible nasolaryngoscopy, again to identify potential primary site
     - Ear examination: Unilateral otitis media with effusion
4. Investigations:
   - USS + core biopsy (will give P16 status + EBV status from a good sample)
   - CT base of skull to diaphragm: To assess degree of adenopathy as well as potential secondary malignancies
   - MRI if in level II–III as high risk of oropharyngeal primary, and 30% better soft tissue delineation
   - PET-CT is management of choice in assessing unknown primary – superior to CT alone, but is not always available
     - Reduces unknown primary diagnosis by 1/3
     - CT not necessary if this is undertaken
     - PET SUV elicits if pathological
     - Indications: Confirmed unknown primary, staging of lymphoma, advanced NPC/hypopharyngeal (T4), N3 nodal status for HNSCC
5. Management:
   - All cancers should be discussed in a multi-disciplinary setting
   - Treatment will be based around patient preference and fitness for surgery
   - Initially a panendoscopy + biopsies:
     - Limited evidence for blind biopsies in yielding diagnosis, but tongue base mucosectomy is an option
     - Targeted biopsies if obvious lesion, otherwise unilateral tonsillectomy should be a minimum

        - Robotic or transoral laser tongue base mucosectomy in available centres is a viable option. Identifies cancers in two-thirds with normal imaging
    - Usually multi-modality treatment:
        - CRT can be offered with salvage procedure, although morbidity may be higher
        - CRT to be offered in all disease from N1 with ECS onwards
        - MRND/SND for all stages except N3
        - Bilateral neck treatment in higher stage disease, i.e. N2–N3
        - Neo-adjuvant CT for those with grossly unresectable disease
            - N1: SND
            - N1 (ECS): SND + RT ± CT
            - N2a/b/c: MRND/SND (±bilateral) + RT (±bilateral) ±CT
            - N3: MRND (type 1) (±bilateral) + RT (±bilateral) ± CT

          (Treatment of the N3 neck is usually non-curative)
        - Key messages:
            - All except N1 get PO(C)RT
            - No evidence that mucosal irradiation improves 5-yr survival or locoregional control
        - A 5-yr follow-up advised, 2 monthly in first 2 years at least, then up to 6 monthly thereafter
        - PET-CT at 3 months post-treatment
6. Differentials:
    - Malignant:
        - Metastatic: HPV/Non-HPV oropharyngeal, thyroid, cutaneous SCC, other head and neck
        - Lymphoma
    - Benign: Reactive LN, branchial cyst, lipoma
7. Evidence:
    - See Farooq et al. Transoral tongue base mucosectomy for identification of primary site in work-up of CUP. Systematic review. Oral Oncol. 2019; 91: 97–106
        - For p16+ tumours
        - Two-thirds of otherwise negative cancers identified by method
        - 5% bleeding rate

Neck Dissection and Terminology

- Neck dissection: Surgical removal of lymph nodes from neck
- Incision depends on:
    - Site of primary
    - Levels treated

  - Uni/bilateral disease
  - Previous scars, relaxed skin tension lines
- Surgical landmarks:
  - Carotid bifurcation: C4
  - Omohyoid
- Radiological landmarks:
  - C4
  - Cricoid
- Nodal levels:

I: Submental, between anterior bellies of digastrics
Submandibular, bound posteriorly by posterior belly of digastric and stylohyoid, anteriorly by the anterior belly of digastric and superiorly by the mandible
II: Skull base superiorly to carotid bifurcation/hyoid
a/b separated by accessory nerve
III: Inferior border of hyoid to inferior border of cricoid
From lateral border of sternohyoid – posterior border of SCM
IV: Inferior border of cricoid to clavicle
V: Posterior triangle:
Bound by posterior border of SCM and anterior border of trapezius
a/b separated by inferior border of cricoid
VI: Including Delphian node
From common carotid artery to common carotid artery in vertical plane, and hyoid to sternal notch in horizontal plane
VII: Below suprasternal notch, but above brachiocephalic artery

- Neck dissection incisions Figure 1.4:
  - Gluck incision:
    - Apron flap + bilateral vertical limbs for supra-clavicular lesions
    - Used for laryngectomy as stoma can be incorporated within apex of apron incision
  - Schobinger:
    - Protects carotid but posteriorly placed flap is prone to devascularisation
  - Conley:
    - Modified Schobinger, with posterior/superior arm brought forward and inferior limb placed postero-laterally (reversal of each limb)
  - Martin: selective ND
    - Double Y as inferior Y allows access to supra-clavicular region
    - S shaped for better cosmesis
    - Two trifurcations means high risk of skin necrosis

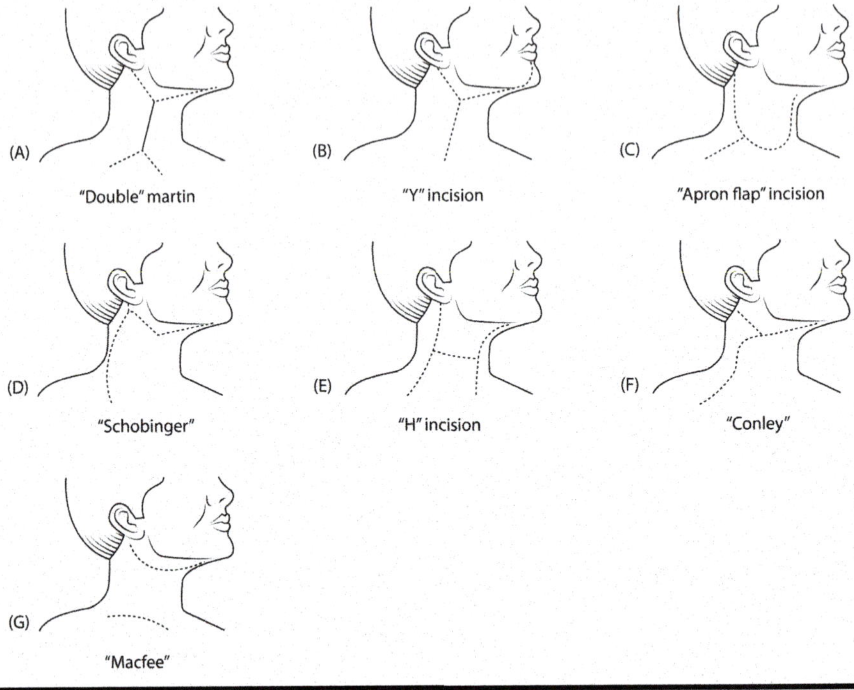

Figure 1.4 Neck dissection incisions.

- MacFee:
  - Parallel incisions
  - Good for cosmesis and blood supply, but poor for access/approach
- ■ Classification of neck dissection:
  - Therapeutic (N+) vs Elective (prophylactic for high-risk pathology – >20% risk of occult disease)
    - Can be undertaken for access for a free flap
  - Radical: All nodal levels (I–V) + CNXI + IJV + SCM
    - Significant morbidity, risk of blowout
    - Low risk of residual disease
    - Indicated in ECS, involvement of structures
  - Extended radical: As above + removal of other levels or structures (VII, XII, levator scapulae, digastric, skin, carotid)
  - Modified radical: As a radical neck dissection but preserving:
    - Type 1) preserving CN XI
    - Type 2) preserving CN XI and IJV
    - Type 3) preserving CN XI, IJV and SCM
      - ■ Technically more difficult but low morbidity
      - ■ Selective (SND): Only removal of high-risk groups

- SND levels I–III (previously known as supra-omohyoid): Oral cavity
  - o SND levels II–IV (previously known as lateral): Oropharynx, hypopharynx, larynx
  - o SND levels II–V (previously known as postero-lateral): Skin/scalp (SCC, melanoma to tragus)
  - o Levels VI (previously known as central): Diff thyroid cancer, subglottic
- Level IIb only excised in N+ disease or in instances of parotid malignancies, oral tongue and hypopharynx cancers. Risk of skeletonising and devascularising accessory nerve leading to dysfunction
- Early risks:
  - General: GA, pain, infection, bleeding, scarring, numbness
  - CN injury (7, 10, 11, 12)
  - Phrenic nerve/brachial plexus injury
  - Horner's syndrome
  - Pneumothorax
  - Stroke
  - Chyle leak
- Late risks:
  - Fistula, wound dehiscence
  - Keloid, hypertrophic scar
- Landmarks for CN XI:
  - 1 cm above Erb's point (emergence of cervical plexus)
  - Deep to posterior belly of digastric
  - Superficial to IJV (80%)
  - SCM tendon

Post-laryngectomy Complications

Chyle leak:

1. Background:
   - Post-neck dissection complication
   - Chyle contains lymphatic fluid and chylomicrons (monoglycerides and fatty acids)
   - Thoracic duct (left lymphatic duct) drains 75% of body
     - Drains at Pirogoff angle (junction between IJV and subclavian)
     - Found in root of neck, posterior and medial to carotid artery and vagus nerve
   - Right lymphatic duct drains right upper quadrant of the body
     - Drains into right subclavian vein

- Chyle leak classified based on output:
  - Low <500 mL/24 hours
  - High >500 mL/24 hours
    - Risks: Dehydration, malnutrition, vessel blowout

2. Investigations:
   - Triglyceride level (>100 mg/dl)
   - Presence of chylomicrons
   - Triglycerides > serum triglycerides
3. Management:
   - Conservative (low output):
     - Bed rest at 45 degrees
     - Reduce activities that raise intrathoracic pressure
     - Medium chain triglyceride diet (absorbed directly into portal system, will reduce output)
   - Medical:
     - Octreotide
     - Total parenteral nutrition
   - Surgical exploration:
     - Oversewing thoracic duct and application of sealant
     - Local muscle flaps
     - VATs-assisted thoracic duct ligation

Pharyngocutaneous fistula:

1. Background:
   - Fistulous tract between pharyngeal mucosa and skin
   - Persistence beyond 4/52 increases risk of vessel blowout
   - Risk factors:
     - Nutritional: Anaemia, low albumin, electrolyte disturbances
     - PMH: Immunocompromise, COPD, hypothyroidism, cardiovascular disease
     - DH: DMARDs, chemotherapy
     - SH: Smoking/alcohol excess
     - Procedure: Salvage surgery, high tumour stage, positive margins, tracheostomy
2. Investigations:
   - Contrast swallow
3. Management:
   - Conservative: NBM, NG or alternative enteral feed, dressings
   - Medical: Antibiotic therapy, hyoscine patch, PPI therapy
   - Surgical:
     - If wound breakdown or vessel exposure:

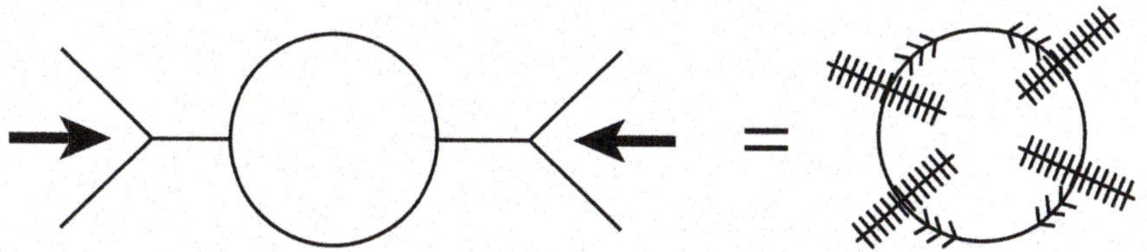

Figure 1.5 The bilateral Y-V inset flap for stomal stenosis.

- Primary closure
- Pec major regional flap
- Free flaps (flaps requiring microvascular anastomosis have higher risk of failure)

Stomal stenosis:

1. Background:
   - Incidence 10–20%
   - Impairs vocalisation
   - Rarely leads to airway compromise
   - Reduced by surgical technique
2. Management:
   - Conservative: Dilatation with laryngectomy tube
   - Surgical:
     - Cartilage split + V-Y inset flap
     - Y-V inset flaps (bilateral – Figure 1.5)

Voice Rehabilitation Post-Laryngectomy

- Types of speech available:
  - Oesophageal:
    - Difficult modality requiring training
    - Process:
      - Air diverted from pharynx into upper oesophagus
      - Upper oesophagus is dilated
      - Air is passed through pharyngo-oesophageal segment (PES) in a controlled manner along with oral manipulation to produce words (five per breath)
      - Voice is typically lower in pitch and more strenuous
    - Vibration of pharyngo-oesophageal sphincter
  - Tracheoesophageal with aid of prosthesis:
    - Secondary puncture undertaken if in salvage or flap presence

- Puncture between posterior tracheal wall and upper oesophagus
- Permits one-way flow (prevents aspiration) into the vibratory PES
- Lifespan of 90 days
- Outer diameter in French sizing, and length usually from 4 to 22 mm. 1 French = 0.33 mm
- Vibration of oesophagus/pharynx (PE) creates noise, which can be modified by oral manipulation to produce voice
  - Primary: At time of surgery
  - Secondary: As a staged procedure following initial surgery (preferred in salvage/post RT setting – Taube air insufflation test)
  - Types: Provox (beveled oesophageal segment) and Blom-Singer have flat flanges
    - Indwelling:
      - Requires expertise to be available locally for changes
      - Utilised where patient dexterity/capabilities are limited (ex-dwelling not feasible)
      - Changed by healthcare professional
    - Non-indwelling (ex-dwelling):
      - Attached safety medallion prevents aspiration
      - Can be changed by patient, although shorter lifespan
- Management of leak/vocalisation issues:
  - Remain NBM until assessment: Use plug as risk of aspiration
  - Consider stomal recurrence as a differential
  - Ensure protection of airway by means of tracheostomy tube (cuffed) if significant leak
  - Assess site of leak:
    - Central: Due to device failure. Clean or swab for Candida. Replace
    - Peripheral: Due to incorrect length or compromised wall. Downsize and encourage stenosis. Increase in size can cause breakdown. Or inject filler. Persistent failure will require removal and reconstruction (very challenging). Removal may encourage stenosis. If not, then TF graft, local or free flaps
    - Consider nasolaryngoscopy to ensure adequate positioning of posterior flange as well as to assess for recurrence (GA)
  - Assess for candida, swab for MC&S and consider nystatin
  - Failed good voice:
    - SALT: Technique and valve type, e.g. high-pressure vs low-pressure
    - Change prosthesis
    - Assess position with nasolaryngoscopy
    - Revise TOP
    - If above fail: Likely PE problem, could be related to RT

        - o Exclude cricopharyngeus muscle stenosis: Dilatation
        - o If no identifiable cause found, consider videofluoroscopy to rule out cricopharyngeal spasm. Revision myotomy or Botox
        - o Oesophageal speech or electrolarynx
    - Key factors in achieving good voice outcomes:
        - ■ A capacious PES
        - ■ A pliable PES to allow sufficient vibration
        - ■ Surgical steps to achieve good voice outcomes:
            - o Tension-free closure of neopharynx
            - o Cricopharyngeal myotomy
            - o Pharyngeal plexus neurectomy
            - o Flattening of lower neck (SCM tenotomy), permits adhesion of base plate and so occlusion for voice and better HME (heat and moisture exchange) filter adhesion
                - – HME filters improve lung function by reducing mucous production and thus suction requirements
                - – One adhesive/baseplate per day is typically used, with 1–2 HME cassettes
                - – Or direct attachment to laryngectomy tube
- – Electrolarynx (Servox, Nu-Voice, Ultravoice):
    - Can be used almost immediately, post-operatively
    - Induces vibrations of the pharyngeal or oral mucosa
    - Oral manipulation modifies vibratory noise into comprehensible speech
    - Are either:
        - ■ Intra-oral (contact with base of tongue, buccal or pharyngeal mucosa):
            - o Less dissipated energy compares to transcutaneous method
            - o Utilised in those with distorted neck anatomy or unable to tolerate pressure
        - ■ Transcutaneous devices

Radiotherapy

1. Background:
    - – Ionising radiation damages cell DNA, resulting in double stranded DNA breaks causing radiation induced reproductive death when cell ready to divide.
    - – Methods:
        - External: Intensity-modulated radiation therapy (IMRT), stereotactic
        - Brachytherapy: Radioiodine, iodine seed implants

- 100 Rads = 1 Gy = Energy/kg = J/kg
- Oxygenated cells more prone to radiation damage
  - Larger tumours = larger hypoxic core = less sensitive
  - Exophytic tumours are more vascularised, hence sensitive to radiation
  - Tumours are most sensitive during mitosis, G1 and S phase (GSM)
- Methods/regime in typical T3 laryngeal Ca:
  - 60–70 Gy/30–35 fractions (primary/radical RT) over 6–7 weeks
  - Prophylactic dose to neck if high risk of occult disease – 50–55 Gy
  - For adjuvant post-operative radiotherapy – 60 Gy in 30 fractions over 6 weeks
- Intensity modulated radiotherapy (IMRT): Dose profile varied to spare normal tissue
- Reasons for fractionation:
  - Opportunity for cells to move into more sensitive stages of cell cycle
  - Allows cells to become recover oxygenation, thus sensitive
  - Normal tissue has time to heal between treatments

2. Indications:
   - Primarily for malignant disease, there are a few benign conditions where radiotherapy is indicated (Table 1.9)
3. Side effects:
   - Can be divided in to systemic (fatigue, lethargy, secondary cancers) and local (Table 1.10)

Table 1.9 Indications for Radiotherapy

Non-Malignant Indications	*Malignant Indications*

• Benign neoplasia: Pituitary adenoma, schwannoma
  • Failed/inoperable juvenile angiofibroma
  • Recurrent pleomorphic adenoma
  • Carotid body tumour
• Keloid scarring
• Grave's eye disease
	• Primary treatment for early-stage disease
	• Concomitant alongside CT
	• Adjuvant: Post-surgery: Higher dose due to scarred tissue
	  • Advanced disease (T or N)
	  • Extracapsular spread
	  • Peri-neural/lymphovascular spread
	  • Involved margins
	• Palliation (metastatic pain or obstructive causes)
	• Alternative types of radiotherapy: Brachytherapy, protons and carbon ions

Table 1.10 Side Effects of Radiotherapy

Side Effects of Radiotherapy
Systemic: • Fatigue/lethargy • Secondary cancers
Laryngeal: • Non-functional larynx (reduced laryngeal elevation, loss of tongue base bolus propulsion, reduced sensation, reduced glottic mobility – aspiration) • Radionecrosis (arytenoid)
GI: • Mucositis, xerostomia, dysphagia (stricture)

OMFS:
• Osteoradionecrosis mandible:
  • Rarely occurs in maxilla, anterior mandible most common
  • Non-healing exposed bone present for 3 months in previously irradiated area
  • Discharge, pain and pathological fractures associated
  • Risks: <50 Gy dose, diabetes, cardiovascular disease, smoking, high-stage disease, dental infection, bisphosphonates
  • Treatment:
    ■ Conservative: Address underlying risk factors and nutrition
    ■ Medical: Hyperbaric oxygen (limited evidence)
    ■ Surgical: Biopsy to exclude recurrence, resection and reconstruction (fibular free flap)

Otological: • SNHL, CHL, tinnitus, persistent ear infection
Ophthalmology: • Cataracts
Impaired healing: • Slow healing • Skin breakdown
Endocrine: • Alopecia, hypothyroidism
Vascular: • Carotid blowout

Chemotherapy

1. Background:
   - Systemic use of chemical agents to treat disease
   - Strategies include neo-adjuvant, concurrent, adjuvant (Table 1.11) and palliative
2. Indications:
   - Nasopharyngeal cancer (advanced stages)
   - Laryngeal organ preservation
   - Unknown primary, particularly if N2–3 disease
   - Recurrence/distant metastasis
   - Unresectable head and neck cancer (palliation)
   - Adjuvant treatment post primary surgical resection if
     - Positive margins
     - Extracapsular disease
3. Agents:
   - A number of agents are used in head and neck cancers (Table 1.12)
     Palliative chemotherapy for unresectable recurrent or metastatic SCC:
     - Assessment of tumour expression of PD-L1 (protein death ligand 1)
     - If the combined positive score (CPS) is 1 or more then pembrolizumab is recommended, that is targeted immunotherapy (targets and blocks protein death 1 protein – PD-1 – in the surface of T-cells. This

Table 1.11 Chemotherapy Strategies

Neo-Adjuvant (Induction)	*Concurrent with Primary Radical RT*	*Concurrently with Adjuvant RT*
• Prior to local treatment (surgery, radiotherapy) • Drug penetration better prior to vascular compromise from RT or surgery • Reduction in tumour bulk enabling controlled resection • More debilitating and possibly increased complications following surgery. • Surgical margins more difficult to assess	• RT + CT now standard for locally advanced cancers of oropharynx, larynx and hypopharynx • Level 1 evidence only for <70-year-olds • CT sensitises cells to RT • Reduction of size of tumour allows improved CT delivery • More debilitating with dual side effect profile	• To control microscopic disease • Multiple nodes, extracapsular spread, positive margins, recurrence • Improves survival

Table 1.12 Chemotherapeutic Agents in H&N Cancer

Platins (alkylating agents): • Cisplatin/carboplatin: • Bind to DNA and RNA • Side effects: Peripheral neuropathy, SNHL, nephrotoxicity • Cisplatin most commonly used in primary and recurrent H&N cancers • Carboplatin better tolerated, not investigated in H&N	**Taxanes:** • Docetaxel/paclitaxel • Prevent normal microtubular re-organisation • Side effects: Neutropenia, alopecia, mucositis • Neo-adjuvant in advanced H&N cancers in combination with 5-FU/ Cisplatin
Anti-metabolites: • 5-FU • Prevents DNA synthesis in S phase • Side effects: Alopecia, mucositis, myelosuppression, cardiotoxicity • Most studied combination with cisplatin in H&N cancer with similar indications	**Monoclonal antibodies (-mab suffix):** • Antibody targeting receptors/ proteins on surface of tumour cells to cause lysis • Cetuximab binds to EGFR and inhibits function and is most commonly used monoclonal chemotherapy in H&N cancer • Can be used where platins contraindicated
Tyrosine kinase inhibitors (-nib suffix): • Targets enzyme responsible for signaling (division/growth) such as RET, MET and VEGF	

prevents the binding and activation of PD-L1. It results in the activation of T-cells against tumour cells. This action would have been otherwise inhibited from the PD-1 to PD-L1 binding). Administration: every 3–6 weeks. Stopped at 2 yrs or earlier if disease progression (NICE guideline – TAA661)

- If CPS <1, cisplatin-based chemotherapy (platinum and 5-FU) is given. For cancer with primary site in the oral cavity, the EXTREME regime is indicated. Cetuximan (eGFR inhibitor) + chemotherapy (platinum and 5-FU. Cetuximab loading dose of 400 mg/m^2 body area, then maintenance dose of 250 mg/m^2 weekly, until disease progression (EXTREME trial, NICE guidance – TA473)
- Nivolumab is recommended when disease progressed after 6 months on platinum-based chemotherapy. It is targeted immunotherapy (human immunoglobulin G4 [IgG4] monoclonal antibody – similar action to pembrolizumab). It is considered a life-extending treatment

at the end of life (up to 9 months longer survival compared to other treatments). Administration: 3 mg/kg every 2 weeks IV over 60 min. Nivolumab is stopped at 2 years or earlier if disease progression (CheckMate 141 trial, NICE Guideline – TA736)

4. Evidence:
   - See Mehanna H et al. Radiotherapy plus cisplatin or cetuximab in low-risk human papillomavirus-positive oropharyngeal cancer (De-ESCALaTE HPV): an open-label randomised controlled phase 3 trial. Lancet. 2019; 393(10166): 51–60
     - Toxicity in cisplatin vs cetuximab alongside radiotherapy:
       - No difference in toxicity
       - Worse 2-yr survival in cetuximab
   - See Mehanna et al. PET-CT surveillance vs neck dissection in advanced H&N cancer. NEJM 2016; 374:1444–1454
     - Management of N2/3 neck:
       - PET-CT surveillance at 12/52 ± ND for residual disease vs planned neck dissection
         - More cost-effective
         - Fewer procedures

Stomal Recurrence

1. Background:
   - Poor prognosis
   - May present as fistula
   - Pre-operative risk factors which increase chance of recurrence:
     - Tumour factors:
       - High T category (cartilage involvement)/N staging (level 4 neck nodes, advanced nodal staging, paratracheal nodes)
       - Subglottic involvement
     - Surgical factors:
       - Pre-treatment tracheostomy increases risk of stomal recurrence by 4-fold
       - Positive resection margins/positive margins in trachea/extracapsular spread
       - Salvage laryngectomy after Radiotherapy
2. History:
   - Onset variable, usually several months following laryngectomy
   - Increasing swelling over stoma with subsequent occlusion
   - Contact bleeding/ulceration/pain/other red flags for cancer
   - Pharyngostomal fistula may represent risk factor for development of recurrence

    - More often than not, it is an early complication due to multiple factors, including:
      - Nutritional deficits
      - Co-morbidities (anaemia, hypothyroidism)
      - Tumour and surgical factors as indicated previously

3. Examination:
   - Full head and neck examination to assess:
     - Stoma
     - Oro and neopharynx
       Both above with flexible nasolaryngoscopy
     - For lymphadenopathy
4. Investigations:
   - USS + FNAC/Biopsy stoma site
   - CT/MRI neck/chest with contrast to assess extent of tumour locally as well as potential distant metastasis (± staging PETCT)
   - EUA and Panendoscopy, for local assessment + diagnosis with biopsy
5. Management:
   - Managed within an MDT setting
   - Always discuss options with patient, who may not agree to further radical surgery
   - Curative intent:
     - Radiotherapy:
       - Only a viable option if not previously been administered (sometimes the recurrence can be outside the previously radiated field and thus can be suitable for RT)
     - Surgery:
       - If adequate surgical margins can be predicted
       - If wrapped around carotids: Not resectable
       - If patient fit for surgery
       - Resection of:
         - Lesion + circumferential margin around stoma
         - Manubrium and medial heads of clavicle
         - New lower stoma formation
         - Excision of diseased skin, nodes ± thyroid
         - If neopharyngectomy + oesophagectomy, consider stomach transposition or free flap
         - Defect closed with regional flap, i.e. pec major
         - Removal of involved lymph nodes ± access to mediastinum
   - Palliative intent: In event of non-resectable disease or distant metastasis:
     - Airway management:
       - Conservative:
         - Tracheostomy tube
         - Humidification

- Medical:
  - Steroids
  - Brachytherapy (iridium-192), palliative radiotherapy: Rarely used
  - Palliative chemotherapy (see "Chemotherapy chapter")
- Surgical:
  - Debulking with CO_2 laser or microdebrider

Sisson criteria for staging:

- Type 1: Superior stomal recurrence
- Type 2: Posterior recurrence (oesophageal)
- Type 3: Inferior recurrence (mediastinal)
- Type 4: Lateral recurrence ± carotid sheath

Chapter 2

Paediatrics

Paula Coyle, Eishaan Bhargava, Adnan Darr, Karan Jolly, Kate Stephenson and Michael Kuo

Contents

DOI: 10.1201/9781003247098-2

Tonsillitis and Post-Tonsillectomy Bleed

1. Background:
   - MALT
   - Waldeyer's ring: Adenoids, lingual/pharyngeal/tubular tonsils
   - Common pathogens:
     - Viral: EBV, CMV, adenovirus, parainfluenza
     - Bacterial: Group A/B/C Streptococcus, bacteroides, fusobacterium
   - Complications of tonsillitis:
     - Abscess formation: Peritonsillar, parapharyngeal, retropharyngeal
     - Lemierre's syndrome: Fusobacterium
     - Systemic: Scarlet fever, rheumatic fever, glomerulonephritis (Streptococcus)
   - Complications of tonsillectomy: Haemorrhage (primary vs secondary), infection, orodental trauma
2. History:
   - Volume of bleed
   - Timing primary (within 24 hrs) vs secondary (>24 hrs post-operatively)
3. Examination (APLS guidance):
   - Airway: Assess signs of stridor/stertor
   - Breathing: Saturations and assess for tachypnoea (aspiration)
   - Circulation: BP, HR and CRT
   - Disability/exposure: GCS, temperature, oropharyngeal examination to identify site of bleed and suction only if obstructive
4. Management:
   - IV access and bloods: U&Es, FBC, CRP, clotting profile, cross match two units
   - IV fluids: 20 mL/kg bolus – normal saline
     - Weight: (Age + 4) × 2
     - Circulating blood volume/kg: 70–75 mL (children), 75–80 mL (infant), 80–85 mL (neonate)
   - Conservative: Sit upright, head tilted forward
   - Medical:
     - Hydrogen peroxide gargles (if tolerated)
     - Adrenaline-soaked gauze to fossa (if tolerated)
     - Tranexamic acid IV
     - Antibiotics

- Surgical (pharyngoscopy + arrest of haemorrhage):
    - Control bleeding: Bipolar cautery → ligation of vessel → surgical + suturing of tonsillar pillars
    - Not controlled with above: Pack oropharynx + transfer intubated to ITU
    - Plan pack removal ± ECA ligation/embolisation if continues to bleed
- Ethical considerations in Jehovah witness:
    - Active bleeding in young child → life-threatening emergency; treat in best interest and transfuse if needed

Blood supply of tonsil:

- Tonsillar branch of facial artery
- Ascending pharyngeal artery
- Ascending palatine artery (facial artery)
- Lesser palatine artery (descending palatine artery from internal maxillary artery)
- Dorsal lingual branch (lingual artery)

Centor criteria for bacterial tonsillitis (3+ diagnostic):

- Exudates
- Fever
- Adenopathy
- Absence of cough

Indications for tonsillectomy:

- OSA
- Asymmetrical tonsillar hypertrophy
- Recurrent tonsillitis (SIGN criteria = 7 episodes/1 yr, 5/yr 2 consecutive years, 3/yr 3 consecutive years)

Grades of shock:

- Grade I: 0–15% alert, mild tachycardia
- Grade II: 15–30% anxious, moderate tachycardia, increased CRT
- Grade III: 30–40% agitated, hypotension, tachycardia, increased RR
- Grade IV: >40% confused, profound hypotension

Paediatric Lymphadenopathy

1. Background:
    - Malignant neoplasia:
        - High suspicion: >2 cm size with no systemic cause; supraclavicular

        - Lymphoma (60%) > rhabdomyosarcoma (30%) > others (thyroid, nasopharyngeal, neuroblastoma, mucoepidermoid, teratomas)
        - Hodgkin's disease (60%) > non-Hodgkin's disease
    - Benign tumours:
        - Schwannoma
        - Salivary gland tumours (pleomorphic adenoma)
        - Thyroid (follicular adenoma)
    - Inflammatory lymphadenopathy:
        - Non-tuberculous mycobacterium (most common: *Mycobacterium avium* intracellular):
            - Overlying skin: Violaceous hue
            - Cervical lymph nodes > parotid/submandibular
            - Treatment: Controversial; influenced by site/stage – conservative/medical/surgical
        - PFAPA: Treated with tonsillectomy
        - Kawasaki disease: Associated with pyrexia, strawberry tongue, fissured lips, conjunctivitis, rash, coronary aneurysms
        - EBV
        - CMV
        - Brucella: Gram negative. Lymphadenopathy and systemic upset. From domesticated animals, through inhalation via breached mucosa, contaminated meat/dairy
        - Bartonella henselae (cat scratch)
2. History:
    - Onset and duration of neck swelling
    - Location, size: Any fluctuation/progression
    - Pain, overlying skin changes
    - Preceding URTI/coryzal illness
    - Systemic symptoms: Fever, weight loss, rigors, night sweats
    - H/O foreign travel/pets
3. Examination:
    - Full head and neck examination to identify a potential focus/primary
        - Neck lump: Site, size, overlying skin, tenderness, mobility, consistency, fluctuation
        - Oropharyngeal examination (tonsil size/asymmetry)
        - FNE if tolerated to assess nasopharynx
    - Systemic examination:
        - Diffuse lymphadenopathy
        - Hepatosplenomegaly
4. Investigations:
    - Serological:
        - EBV, CMV, Toxoplasma, Bartonella, FBC, ESR, CRP, LDH
    - Radiological:

        - CXR: Mediastinal nodes or metastatic spread (rhabdomyosarcoma/thyroid or salivary gland malignancy)
        - USS ± needle biopsy (role of needle biopsy vs excisional biopsy controversial; consider in older children/when high surgical risk with whole node excision):
            - Cluster of nodes, architecture and proximity to vascular structures
            - Abnormal if round, loss of fatty hilum, peripheral flow, >1 cm long axis
        - CT neck/thorax/abdomen/pelvis if high index of suspicion of lymphoma
    - Surgical:
        - Incisional/excisional biopsy
5. Management:
    - Conservative wait and watch: For suspected reactive nodes, with no adverse features on USS
    - Medical management: Dependent on infectious aetiology
    - Paediatric oncology MDT involvement following collation of investigations if suspected malignancy to guide need for surgical intervention

Differential diagnosis of paediatric lateral neck mass:

- Congenital: Branchial cleft anomaly
- Infection: See inflammatory lymphadenopathy causes
- Benign neoplasia: Schwannoma, salivary gland neoplasm, thyroid neoplasm, lymphatic malformation
- Malignant neoplasia: Lymphoma, rhabdomyosarcoma, thyroid neoplasm, metastatic neck secondary

Otitis Media with Effusion

1. Background:
    - Peak incidence 2–5 yrs, resolved by 8–10 yrs
    - Aetiopathology:
        - Eustachian tube dysfunction/obstruction results in negative middle ear pressure due to absorption/diffusion of nitrogen and oxygen into middle ear cleft mucosal cells
        - If negative pressure sufficient, will result in formation of transudate from mucosa
2. History:
    - Subjective hearing loss: Duration, fluctuation/persistent
    - Delayed speech and language development
    - Poor educational progression/behavioural concerns
    - Balance problems/clumsiness

  - Recurrent infections (AOM/URTI)
  - H/O risk factors (see text)
3. Examination:
  - Adenoidal facies: Open mouth, long face, high-arched palate
  - Otoscopy
  - Assessment for adenoidal hypertrophy: Cold spatula test; FNE
  - Syndromic features
4. Investigations:
  - Audiometry (age-appropriate)
  - Tympanometry
5. Management:
  - Conservative:
    - Purely observational: 50% resolve at 3 months and 90% at 12 months
    - Autoinflation
    - Hearing aids: Surgery is declined or trisomy 21/cleft palate
  - Surgical:
    - Grommets: If meeting following criteria:
      - Bilateral glue ear + 25–30-dB HL in better hearing ear averaged at 0.5, 1, 2, 4 kHz following 3-month period of observation
    - Possible role of adjuvant adenoidectomy alongside revision grommets in persistent OME – weigh risks against potential benefits
    - Risks of procedure:
      - Otorrhoea (8%)
      - Perforation (4%)
      - Early extrusion
  - Following are NOT indicated in OME:
    - Long-term antibiotics
    - Topical (nasal)/oral antihistamines
    - Topical (nasal) steroids
    - Homeopathy, cranial osteopathy or acupuncture
6. Evidence:
  - Cochrane Database (2016): Antibiotics in OME
    - Moderate evidence for resolution of glue at 2–3 months
    - No evidence suggesting fewer ventilation tube insertions, hearing/speech/language or cognitive improvement
  - Cochrane Database (2013): Autoinflation in OME
    - Small cohort, short-term period evaluated, but low cost and morbidity suggest autoinflation as a viable option
  - Cochrane Database (2010): Adenoidectomy in OME (chronic or acute)
    - Resolution of OME, minimal benefit on hearing, but must weigh up risks against benefits
  - TARGET study (2012): Adjuvant adenoidectomy in persistent OME – better hearing, reduced need for revision surgery

Risk factors

Patient:
- Craniofacial abnormalities: Syndromic; cleft palate
- Primary ciliary dyskinesia/cystic fibrosis
- Atopy/recurrent URTI

Environmental:
- Passive smoking
- Low socio-economic group
- Bottle feeding
- Siblings in school
- Nursery attendance
- Seasonal

NICE: Trisomy 21
- Avoid grommets (difficult access + anaesthetic risks)
- Hearing aid first line → grommets (mini-Shah)

NICE: Cleft palate
- Hearing aid first line where possible
- Grommets to be considered at the time of palate repair, if indicated

Acute Otitis Media

1. History:
   - Recent coryzal symptoms/URTI
   - Otalgia, otorrhea, imbalance, hearing loss
   - Facial weakness
   - Systemic: Fever, headaches, erratic behaviour
   - Previous bouts of AOM
   - PMH: h/s/o immunodeficiency
   - Vaccination history
2. Examination:
   - Pinna position, post-auricular region – r/o mastoiditis
   - Otoscopy: Bulging erythematous tympanic membrane/perforated tympanic membrane with blood-stained discharge
   - Facial nerve examination
3. Investigations:
   - Audiometry/tympanometry
   - CT with contrast first line in event of suspected complication
4. Management:
   - NICE guidelines
     - 3 days observation if not systemically unwell
     - Systemically unwell/no improvement in 3 days → oral antibiotics

        - Exceptions:
            - Febrile child <3 month → immediate inpatient treatment
            - Signs of complication → immediate inpatient treatment
            - Any child <2 yrs → oral antibiotics first line
    - Myringotomy and grommet rarely indicated:
        - Complications, including facial nerve palsy
        - No improvement despite medical management
        - Recurrent AOM

5. Evidence:
    - Cochrane Database (2018): Grommets in AOM:
        - Low-quality evidence suggests reduction in number of episodes prior to pneumococcal vaccination
    - Cochrane Database (2015): Antibiotics in the use of AOM
        - Around 1/14 adverse events from antibiotics
        - Limited role, in children under 2 yrs of age

Pathogens:

- Viral:
    - RSV
    - Rhinovirus
    - Adenovirus
    - Parainfluenza virus
- Bacterial:
    - *Streptococcus pneumoniae*
    - *Haemophilus influenzae*
    - *Moraxella catarrhalis*

Risk factors:

- Environmental
    - Passive smoking
    - Low socio-economic status
    - Nursery
    - No breastfeeding
    - Dummy use
- Host:
    - A period of 3 months to 3 yrs
    - Male
    - Family history: Siblings
    - Craniofacial abnormality
    - Primary ciliary dyskinesia/cystic fibrosis
    - Immunodeficiency
    - Gastro-oesophageal reflux

Complications of Acute Otitis Media

1. Background:
   - Routes of spread:
     - Haematogenous/lymphatic through venous channels
     - Local erosion of bone/osteitis (tegmen defects)
     - Fracture lines/bony defects/fissures of Santorini
     - Normal structures: Round/oval window
2. History:
   - History of preceding URTI and OME or ongoing otorrhoea
   - Fluctuating pyrexia (swinging)
   - Meningism: Triad of neck stiffness, headache (cavernous sinus thrombosis, IC abscess) and photophobia
   - Irritability and mental status change (low GCS)
3. Examination:
   - ABCDE approach
   - ENT:
     - Otoscopy will demonstrate a bulging erythematous tympanic membrane/blood-stained otorrhoea with perforation
     - Mastoid swelling
   - Neurological:
     - GCS
     - Assess for meningism
     - Kernig's (neck flexion on hip flexion and passive knee extension) and Brudzinski's signs (hip flexion on neck flexion)
     - Cranial nerves: Facial nerve or abducens nerve weakness
4. Investigations:
   - IV access, CRP, FBC, blood cultures and lactate
   - CT scan of temporal bones + brain with contrast
     - Indications:
       - Preoperative planning
       - No improvement following 48 hrs of antibiotics
       - Mastoid abscess
       - Neurological symptoms (CN palsy, reduced GCS, meningism)
       - Swinging pyrexia (CST)/systemic upset
5. Management:
   - Medical:
     - Antibiotics, as per trust anti-microbial guidelines (third-generation cephalosporin such as ceftriaxone), IV fluids (20 mL/kg saline) and strict urine output chart
     - Anticoagulation to prevent clot propagation (dependent on local haematology guidelines): 3 months of Warfarin, with re-scan, and if no further propagation, can discontinue

- Surgical: Managed in a multidisciplinary setting with ENT and neurosurgical input:
  - Minimum EUA ears, myringotomy + grommet + cortical mastoidectomy with swabs + washout + drain
  - Post-operative transfer to ITU or neurosurgical unit

6. Evidence:
   - Cochrane 2011: Anticoagulation for cerebral venous sinus thrombosis:
     - Limited data. Safe with reduction in mortality. Not statistically significant. No data for paediatric population
   - See Wong et al. Management of otogenic paediatric CVST: A systematic review. Clin Otol 2015; 40(6): 704–714
     - Good outcome with combination surgery and anticoagulation

Complications of AOM

- Intracranial: (*Streptococcus milleri*)
  - Meningitis
  - Abscess:
    - Temporal lobe abscess
    - Extradural abscess
    - Subdural abscess
  - Otic hydrocephalus
  - Lateral sinus thrombosis
- Extracranial:
  - Intra-temporal:
    - Labyrinthitis
    - Facial nerve palsy
    - Gradenigo syndrome (petrous apicitis – triad of retro-orbital pain, CN 6 palsy and otorrhoea)
    - Mastoiditis
  - Extra-temporal (abscesses)
    - Bezold's abscess (SCM from mastoid)
    - Citelli (posterior belly digastric from mastoid)
    - Luc's abscess (Zygomatic)
    - Subperiosteal
- Systemic:
  - Embolic spread

Choanal Atresia

1. Background:
   - Aetiology:
     - Persistence of buccopharyngeal membrane

    - Failure of bucconasal membrane rupture
    - Medial outgrowth of horizontal and vertical portions of palatine bone
  - Unilateral > bilateral (2:1), Rt (65%) > Lt, F>M
  - Bony (30%), mixed (70%), membranous (rare)
  - Bony from lateral pterygoid plates and medial from vomer
  - Associations (in 50% of cases):
    - CHARGE syndrome
    - 22q11 deletion syndrome
    - Craniosynostosis syndromes with early fusion: Crouzon and Apert
    - Treacher Collins syndrome
    - Down's (trisomy 21) and Edward's syndromes (trisomy 18)
2. History:
   - Unilateral: Rhinorrhoea, congestion, anosmia, which may not be detected for years
   - Bilateral:
     - Neonatal airway emergency
     - Cyclical cyanosis with neonatal respiratory distress due to obligate nasal respiration alleviated when crying
3. Examination:
   - Anterior rhinoscopy and nasal flow assessment (wisp of cotton/cold spatula test/stethoscope)
   - Inability to pass fine bore feeding tube or 8F catheter on affected side
   - FNE
   - Syndromic features
4. Investigations:
   - Genetic testing: CHD7 gene in CHARGE
   - Cardiac screening (echo/ECG)
   - Renal USS
   - CT (gold standard), to assess following:
     - Confirmation of diagnosis
     - Type of atresia (membranous, bony or mixed)
     - Evaluate bony aspect (vomer width and choanal distance)
   - Rhinogram
5. Management:
   - Airway: Oropharyngeal airway/intubation (where oropharyngeal airway ineffective)
   - Conservative: Use of McGovern nipple for feeds
   - Medical: Orogastric feed/supplementation until surgical correction is undertaken
   - Early surgical correction:
     - Endoscopic transnasal approach:
       - ■ Curette with posterior membranous flap covering bone. Powered instrumentation may be needed

        - Endoscopic retropalatal (transoral) approach:
            - ■ Advantageous as less room in newborn to use endoscope in nasal cavity
            - ■ Tonsil/cleft gag utilised, with Draffin rods and 120-degree scope
            - ■ Urethral dilators/Hegar dilators utilised to puncture atretic plate (membranous component is infero-medial usually)
            - ■ Medial pterygoid plates can be drilled, and vomer resected
        - Transpalatal:
            - ■ Not recommended due to effect of growth of maxilla, increased operative time, blood loss, fistulation, VPI
    - Post-operative saline, decongestant and steroid drops
    - Stent:
        - Varied practice across the UK – no consensus
        - No strong evidence of decreased risk of stenosis
        - Complications of stenting: Blocking, columellar necrosis, alar notching, infection, ulceration, granulation tissue formation and circumferential scarring
    - Risks of surgery: Restenosis, midfacial growth arrest (vomer resection), saddling, skull-base injury
6. Differential diagnoses:
    - Structural: Nasal pyriform aperture stenosis, deflected/dislocated nasal septum, dacrocystocoele
    - Mucosal: Neonatal rhinitis, mucosal swelling, turbinate hypertrophy
    - Neoplasia: Glioma, chordoma, teratoma, encephalocele
7. Evidence:
    - Cochrane Database (2012): No evidence to suggest benefit of one surgical procedure over another
    - Cochrane Database (2015) Meta-analysis: Stents do not prevent restenosis and are associated with complications (septal necrosis, synechiae and displacement)

CHARGE syndrome:

- ■ CHD7 gene
- ■ Coloboma
- ■ Heart defects
- ■ Atresia (choanal) (50% bilateral)
- ■ Retardation of growth
- ■ Genitourinary abnormalities
- ■ Ear abnormalities (Mondini, enlarged vestibular aqueduct, semicircular canal abnormalities)

Primary Ciliary Dyskinesia

1. Background:
    - 50% of PCD patients have Kartagener's syndrome
    - Autosomal recessive
    - Mutations on DNAI1 and DNAH5 genes
    - Structural defects of outer/inner dynein arms (normal arrangement = nine outer pairs + one central pair)
    - Lack a central pair of B and A microtubule doublets which are cross-linked with nexin
    - Structural defect → subsequent altered ciliary beat frequency (normal – 7–22/s or 1000–1500/min) OR orientation → poor mucous clearance → recurrent infections + chronic inflammation (bronchiectasis) (*Haemophilus influenzae* most common organism)
2. Differential diagnoses:
    - Kartagener's syndrome: Variant of PCD
        - Triad of rhinosinusitis, situs inversus, bronchiectasis
    - Young's syndrome: Rhinosinusitis infertility syndrome
    - Cystic fibrosis:
        - Defective chloride transporter CFTR, due to F508 deletion
        - Sweat test chloride levels: <30 (normal), 30–60 (probable) and >60–90 mEq/l almost diagnostic (rule of 30)
            - Pilocarpine can be used to stimulate sweat
        - Delayed meconium passage
        - Malabsorption and COPD
        - Bilateral nasal polyps
        - Pseudomonas most common organism in sinus, unlike PCD (*H. influenzae*)
        - Life expectancy 50 yrs
        - Treatment with Azithromycin for long term, pancreatic enzyme replacement and bronchodilators
        - Surgical treatment for polyposis: High risk of recurrence; indicated in persistent obstruction, fungal infections and exacerbation of respiratory disease
3. History:
    - Most common symptom: Profuse rhinorrhoea
    - Anosmia
    - Nasal obstruction
    - Hearing loss/ear infections
    - Infertility
4. Examination:
    - Nasal polyposis/discharge
    - Glue ear

5. Investigations:
   - Nasal nitric oxide levels in patients >5 yrs
   - Saccharin test: Place 1 cm posterior to head of inferior turbinate → >10–20 min requires referral (not routinely used)
   - Can also use methylene blue in place of saccharin → visualising oropharynx for staining to assess clearance
   - Nasal/bronchial brush biopsies
   - CT sinuses (sinusitis)/chest (bronchiectasis in HRCT)
6. Management:
   - Multidisciplinary approach due to widespread system involvement
   - Genetic counselling
   - Conservative:
     - Chest physiotherapy
     - Nasal douching
     - Autoinflation
   - Medical:
     - Antibiotics for recurrent infections
     - HiB/pneumococcal vaccination
     - Mucolytics
     - Bronchodilators
     - Steroids (oral)
   - Surgical:
     - Ventilation tubes
     - ESS
     - Lung transplantation

Juvenile Nasopharyngeal Angiofibroma

1. Background:
   - Exclusively found in post-pubescent males; hormonal aetiology suggested
   - Originates on lateral nasal wall near sphenopalatine foramen
   - Blood vessel walls lack smooth muscle (muscularis) and elastic fibres, fibrous stroma, hence unable to go into vasospasm
   - Supplied by internal maxillary artery
   - Patients with familial adenomatous polyposis have a 25 times greater risk of having a JNA
2. History:
   - Age (typically adolescent male)
   - Unilateral nasal obstruction
   - Unilateral epistaxis: Laterality, duration, first-aid measures
   - Unilateral hearing loss (glue ear)
   - Headaches and neurological symptoms (visual compromise)

3. Examination:
   - Nasal flow, anterior rhinoscopy, careful FNE (well-circumscribed, smooth lobulated mass, purple/red hue)
   - AVOID probing/rigid endoscopic examination
   - Head and neck examination:
     - Facial swelling if pterygopalatine fossa involved
     - Globe displacement in ethmoid involvement
     - Deformity of nasal bones
4. Investigations:
   - Cross-sectional imaging:
     - Digital subtraction angiography for embolisation
     - CT with contrast paranasal sinuses/head:
       - Anterior bowing of posterior maxillary wall (Holman-Miller sign)
       - Widening of sphenopalatine foramen
     - MRI:
       - Salt and pepper appearance on T2 (due to flow voids)
       - Soft-tissue evaluation/extension:
         - Intracranial, orbit, pterygopalatine fossa
5. Management:
   - Avoid biopsy
   - Conservative: Only for those not fit for surgery
   - Medical (no conservative strategies as aggressive tumour):
     - Hormonal therapy with testosterone receptor blocker (flutamide) or oestrogen, may reduce vascularity and size (adjunct)
     - Radiotherapy: Residual tumours due to secondary malignancy risk, and inoperable tumours extending into skull base
   - Surgical:
     - Preoperative embolisation (24–72 hrs prior): For vessels >2 mm in size
       - Risk of stroke, visual loss, facial pain, cranial nerve neuropathies (rarely)
       - May obscure boundaries, hence increased risk of residual tissue
       - Risk of rendering tumour radioresistant due to hypoxia
     - Endoscopic surgery: Dependent on lateral extent of tumour; associated with similar rate of recurrence but less blood loss than open
     - Open surgery:
       - Lateral rhinotomy, Caldwell-Luc
       - Advanced disease by midfacial degloving or craniofacial resection
       - Basisphenoid region should be drilled out to prevent recurrence
   - Surveillance: Baseline MRI at 6/12 then annually. Highest recurrence 12–24/12

Differential diagnoses:

- Benign:
  - Nasal polyposis/antrochoanal polyp
  - Inverted papilloma
  - Cavernous haemangioma
  - Pyogenic granuloma (if small)
- Malignant:
  - Rhabdomyosarcoma
  - Nasopharyngeal carcinoma (unlikely)
  - Lymphoma

Fisch classification:

I: Nasal cavity, no bony destruction
II: Invading pterygopalatine fossa, paranasal sinuses; negligible bony destruction
III: Invading infratemporal fossa/orbit
  a. Without intracranial involvement
  b. Intracranial extradural involvement
IV: a. Intracranial, intradural
  b. Cavernous sinus/optic nerve involvement

Midline Nasal Mass

1. Background:
   - Dermoid (nasal):
     - Found in areas of embryological fusion
       - Defective obliteration of dural tissue
         - Dura projects through fonticulus nasofrontalis to skin, then retracts. Connection can remain to dura
       - May contain mesoderm or ectodermal components (teratoma contains all three germ layers)
       - Can be intra- or extranasal, or intracranial
       - IC extension in up to 45%
     - Encephalocele:
       - Failure of neural tube closure, thus herniation of cranial contents
       - CSF filled due to communication with subarachnoid space
       - Meningocele (meninges), meningoencephalocele (meninges and brain)
       - Furstenberg sign positive, transilluminates, pulsatile
       - Sincipital (front of head; hence naso-frontal, naso-orbital, naso-ethmoidal)

  - ■ Basal (skull base; hence transethmoidal, sphenoethmoidal, transsphenoidal)
    - o Transethmoidal most common
- Nasal glioma:
  - ■ Purple/blue hue
  - ■ Usually paramedian and on glabella
  - ■ Non-compressible
  - ■ Intranasal (30%), extranasal (60%)
  - ■ Dysplastic glial cells that have lost intracranial connections
  - ■ Fibrous stalk to dura but no communication with dural spaces (unlike encephalocele)

2. History:
   - Timing (from birth, recent increase in size)
   - Exacerbating features (enlargement when crying or straining = encephalocele/meningoencephalocele)
   - Nasal congestion (intranasal aspect)
   - History of meningitis/clear nasal discharge
3. Examination:
   - Nasal flow, anterior rhinoscopy, FNE (intranasal component)
   - Inspection:
     - Pulsation
     - Punctum/hair: Pathognomonic of dermoid
   - Signs:
     - Furstenberg sign (compression of ipsilateral JV causes increase in size) = encephalocele/meningoencephalocele
     - Increase in size on Valsalva
     - Transillumination
4. Investigations:
   - Beta-2-transferrin if rhinorrhoea
   - CT head:
     - Bifid crista galli
     - Dural connection
   - MRI:
     - MRI for soft-tissue delineation as well as diagnosis of hydrocephalus (localise stalk of encephalocele)
5. Management: Mainly surgical, which minimises risk of meningitis
   - MDT, with neurosurgical input if intracranial component
   - Dermoid:
     - Incision/approach: Midline (horizontal or vertical), lateral rhinotomy, brow incision, external septorhinoplasty approach
     - Bicoronal flap and craniotomy for dural extension
   - Encephalocele:
     - ±Fluorescein

- ±Lumbar drain to prevent recurrence due to increased pressure
- Frontal craniotomy (60–80% success rates)
  - ■ Superior visualisation
  - ■ Ideal for repair following acute trauma
  - ■ Disadvantages:
    - o External scar and need for osteotomies
    - o Risk of haemorrhage and anosmia
- Endoscopic approach:
  - ■ Lower morbidity, but not utilised if patient <5 yrs and limited by size of defect
  - ■ Repairs usually need to be robust, hence "gasket-seal" utilised:
    - o Dead space plugged with fat
    - o Fascia lata, 1 cm larger circumferentially
    - o Vomer/inferior turbinate bone to tightly seal bony defect in exact dimension (cartilage weaker)
    - o Mucosal graft overlay invariably also utilised in, for example, irradiated patients:
      - – Nasoseptal flap: Posterior septal branch of SPA
      - – Middle turbinate flap: Middle turbinate artery brand of SPA
      - – Inferior turbinate: Posterior lateral nasal artery from SPA

– Glioma:
- Endoscopically excised if intranasal
- Skin incision if extranasal
- Endoscopic if internal

Differential diagnoses:

- ■ Dermoid
- ■ Glioma
- ■ Encephalocele/meningoencephalocele

Acute Epiglottitis

1. Background:
   - – Commonly seen in 2–4 yr olds in pre-HiB vaccination era
   - – Mortality approaches 6%
   - – Complications include:
     - Sepsis

  - Epiglottic abscess/deep neck space infection
  - Vocal cord granuloma

2. History:
   - Preceding common URTI
   - Rapid onset and progression of symptoms with systemic compromise
   - Rapidly progressing to dysphagia and odynophagia
   - Muffled/hot potato voice
   - Associated with drooling
   - Respiratory effort and distress
   - Stridor (inspiratory) (late sign)
3. Examination:
   - Septic-looking individual, with tachycardia, potential hypotension, tachypnoea, pyrexia
   - Increased work of breathing in tripod position (upright on both hands, with head forward and tongue protruding)
   - Avoid agitating patient, as this may precipitate laryngospasm
   - Adopt APLS ABCDE approach:
     - Transfer to Resus, and inform theatres and on call anaesthetist/ITU team of impending airway compromise
       - ■ Request a tracheostomy set, varied ETT (Age/4)+4), and age appropriate ventilating bronchoscopes
     - Airway: Assess for stridor, position of tongue, drooling, fullness in voice. Avoid use of tongue depressor. If suspected epiglottitis, consider nebulised adrenaline (1 mL of 1:1000, made up to 5 mL with saline) and oral dexamethasone (0.15–0.3 mg/kg)
     - Breathing: Wafting oxygen in the event of tachypnoea and desaturation. Avoid use of face mask
     - Circulation: Assess for tachycardia but avoid use of blood pressure cuff
     - Disability:
       - ■ Temperature and GCS. A reduced GCS coupled with declining parameters may be indicative of impending respiratory arrest
       - ■ Neck examination may yield a tender larynx and adenopathy
4. Investigations:
   - Investigations in the immediate period are avoided as condition is time critical, UNLESS STABLE
   - A chest radiograph may demonstrate thumbprinting (epiglottis ≥7 mm thick) as well as obliteration of vallecula (vallecula sign)
   - Once the airway has been secured:
     - Swab epiglottis
     - IV access, IV antibiotics as per local protocol (usually third-generation cephalosporin)
     - Blood cultures, FBC, CRP, U&Es, LFTs and clotting

5. Management:
   - Within theatre environment
   - Child managed in an upright position
   - Inhalation anaesthetic used (avoid muscle relaxants)
   - Patient positioned supine, and anaesthesia deepened with spontaneous respiration
   - Solitary attempt is usually made at orotracheal intubation, with the use of a bougie due to further swelling from repeated attempts
   - If orotracheal intubation fails, MLB set-up is used with ETT sheathed on a 4 mm rigid endoscope using a Parsons laryngoscope
     - Alternatively, can use an age-appropriate ventilating bronchoscope
   - Post-operative CXR
   - Transfer to PICU
   - Tube removal when leak noted with cuff deflated
     - Ideally, FNE should be undertaken prior to all extubations

Common organisms

- *Haemophilus influenzae* (less common now due to vaccination)
- *Streptococcus pneumoniae*/viridans
- *Staphylococcus aureus*
- *Aspergillus* (if immunocompromised)

Differential diagnoses:

- Peritonsillar abscess
- Deep neck space infection
- Laryngotracheobronchitis
- Angioedema
- Caustic ingestion
- Supraglottitis

Laryngeal Papillomatosis

1. Background:
   - Typical age of presentation: 3–5 yrs (peak). Younger presentation = more aggressive disease
   - Dysphonia (most common presentation) > stridor (second most common) > respiratory distress
   - 6, 11 most common strain, 11 more aggressive
   - 3% risk of malignancy
   - Tracheal spread associated with higher malignancy rate
   - Most common site in upper airway = glottis, mainly anterior commissure

- Pulmonary involvement rare. Appear as pulmonary cavitating lesions on CT
    - Can result in abscesses and pulmonary haemorrhage
- Vaccination programme (bi- or quadrivalent):
    - Gardasil: 6, 11, 16, 18 strains. In 2019 offered to 12–13 yr olds up until 25th birthday (cervical, head and neck and anogenital)
    - Cervarix: 16 and 18 strains only

2. History:
    - Dysphonia
    - Stridor
    - Exertional dyspnoea
    - Birth history: Mode of delivery and parity
    - PMH: Immunosuppression (flare of previously treated disease)
3. Examination:
    - Head and neck examination
    - FNE within a clinic setting if permitted by patient
    - Evaluated using the Derkay score (subjective scoring system):
        - Clinical evaluation: Voice, stridor, need for surgery and dyspnoea
        - Anatomical: No lesion, surface, raised or bulky
4. Investigations:
    - MLB for diagnosis + excision + histology during first procedure + regular endoscopies for recurrence
5. Management:
    - Conservative: For limited disease, observation with SLT input for voice
    - Adjunctive medical therapy: If >4 surgical procedures/year OR distal tracheal disease
        - Alpha-interferon: Does not eradicate virus, and treatment is usually 6-month period
            - Bone marrow suppression and deranged LFTs
            - No longer used
        - Intralesional cidofovir: Prevents viral replication, inhibition of DNA polymerase
            - Every 4–6 months
            - 5% malignancy risk
            - For limited disease
        - Bevacizumab (Avastin): VEGFR inhibitor, targeting the vascular supply to papillomas
            - SE: Infertility, renal compromise, hypotension
            - Consider for diffuse disease
        - Gardasil also postulated to increase interval between procedures
    - Surgical methods:
        - If anterior commissure involvement, consider staged procedure to prevent webbing
        - Cold steel: Higher scarring rates

- Microdebrider (2.9-mm skimmer blade)
- CO_2 laser: Associated with scarring (sulcus vocalis) and airway fires
- Tracheostomy: A last resort due to risk of distal airway seeding. More an association rather than causation, due to likely aggressive disease

6. Differential diagnoses (paediatric):
   - Chronic laryngitis
   - Vocal cord nodules
   - Vocal cord polyps

Risk factors:

- Mother <20 yrs (low socio-economic status)
- Maternal genital warts
- Vaginal delivery (vertical transmission)
- Prolonged labour: First born

Drooling (Sialorrhea)

1. Background:
   - 1–1.5 l of saliva produced daily, of which 70% of resting saliva is produced by submandibular gland
   - Can be anterior or posterior (usually associated with coughing and symptoms of aspiration)
   - Normal in children ≤24 months, prior to development of oral neuromuscular control. Abnormal if >4 yrs of age
   - Neurological pathology may delay neuromuscular control until 6 yrs of age
2. History:
   - Onset and progression: Sudden (foreign body) or gradual progression
   - Systemic features indicative of potential inflammatory pathology
   - Associated dysphagia of liquids or solids (neurological)
   - Severity (number of bib or clothing changes, perioral rash)
   - PMH: Perinatal history, cerebral palsy, developmental delay
3. Examination:
   - Head positioning/control may demonstrate an underlying neurological disorder
   - Oral/oropharynx:
     - Condition of perioral skin
     - Oral candidiasis, gingivitis, caries
     - Macroglossia and tonsil size/mouth breathing may indicate adenoidal pathology
   - Nasal: Flow (adenoidal pathology)

4. Investigations:
   - FNE if tolerated to assess for adenoidal as well as laryngeal/hypopharyngeal pathology
   - SLT assessment:
     - Contrast swallow: Motility/spasm
     - Videofluoroscopy/FEES: Real-time swallow assessment
5. Management:
   - MDT approach: ENT, neurodisability, SLT, dentists, physical therapist
   - Conservative: Usually 6-month period:
     - Postural changes
     - Behavioural therapy: Positive reinforcement
     - Oral motor therapy/exercises to aid with initial phase of swallowing such as head stability, lip closure and jaw stability
   - Medical:
     - PPI therapy
     - Anticholinergics inhibit activity of muscarinic receptors to reduce volume but can lead to constipation, urinary retention (Hyoscine transdermal 0.5 mg/kg, max 5 mg), Glycopyrrolate (0.1 mg/kg TDS)
     - Botulinum toxin inhibits pre-synaptic release of ACh and thus can also block cholinergic parasympathetic secretomotor fibres to the submandibular gland
       - Usually injected into parotid as well as submandibular glands
     - Radiotherapy: Rarely used treatment due to risk of secondary malignancies
   - Surgical: Undertaken after the age of 6 yrs and usually after failure of or adjunctive to conservative/medical therapy:
     - Adenoidectomy for hypertrophy
     - Tympanic neurectomy (transtympanic = TM flap + division of tympanic plexus on promontory): 50–80% success rate – not commonly used
     - Wharton's ductal re-routing:
       - Not recommended in neurological patients, due to the risk of aspiration due to increased burden on the hypopharynx
       - Rhomboid segment dissected, including both ductal openings, then divided in midline. Duct dissected for 3–4 cm until lingual nerve bisects
       - Submucosal tunnel is made posterior to the anterior pillar, and island is sutured and anterior opening is closed
       - Sublingual gland is excised to minimise ranula formation
       - Complications include a ranula
     - Submandibular gland excision for those who aspirate
     - Parotid duct ligation/2–4 duct ligation/staged multiple duct ligation – adjunct to above methods

Aetiology:

- Excess production, also deemed primary sialorrhoea:
  - Inflammatory: Candidiasis, gingivitis, dental caries, tonsillitis
  - Medication-induced, also deemed secondary:
    - Tranquilisers
    - Anti-cholinesterases
    - Anti-epileptics
  - Systemic:
    - Neurological: Cerebral palsy
    - Gastrointestinal: GORD
- Inability to retain saliva within oral cavity – poor oral-motor control, malocclusion, macroglossia
- Impaired swallowing
  - Neurological: CP, Down's, neuromuscular weakness
  - Anatomical

Preauricular Sinus

1. Background:
   - Lateral and superior to the facial nerve and parotid
   - Inherited in autosomal dominant fashion (20–30% of cases), mainly sporadic
   - Bilateral in 25–50% of cases
   - Due to incomplete fusion of hillocks of His
   - Pits extend to cartilage, sinuses down to tympanic ring
   - Almost always connects to perichondrium of ear cartilage
   - Associations: First arch anomalies
     - Branchio-oto-renal syndrome
     - Goldenhar syndrome
     - Treacher Collins syndrome
2. History:
   - Recurrent infections, ulceration and cellulitis
   - Discharge
   - Abscesses
3. Examination:
   - Indentation/pit ascending limb of helix
   - Otoscopy: Rule out first arch anomaly
4. Investigations:
   - Not routinely investigated
   - Audiometric testing
   - Renal USS to rule out branchio-oto-renal syndrome as a precaution (not routine unless bilateral cleft anomalies)

5. Management:
   - MDT approach
   - Genetic counselling
   - Conservative:
     - Purely observational if asymptomatic
   - Medical:
     - Oral antibiotics for acute infections
   - Surgical:
     - Avoid incision and drainage as they will result in difficulties with eventual excision (consider aspiration)
     - Use of methylene blue or lacrimal probe to delineate tract
     - Elliptical incision of skin
     - Tract dissected with excision of segment of cartilage to prevent recurrence
     - Distal ligation with tie and division at level of temporalis fascia
     - Revision procedure – consider facial nerve monitoring
     - Increased risk of recurrence in the following circumstances:
       - Revision procedure
       - Previous incision and drainage
       - Local anaesthetic procedure
       - Cartilage not excised
       - Simple sinusectomy (50% recurrence rate)
6. Differential diagnoses:
   - Epidermal inclusion cyst
   - First cleft anomaly (See Work et al. XLII The Otologist and First Branchial Cleft Anomalies. Ann Otol Rhinol Laryngol 1963; 72(2), https://doi.org/10.1177/000348946307200221)

Six hillocks of His (first 1–3 and second branchial arches 4–6 at 6 weeks gestation):

- Tragus
- Helical crus
- Helix
- Anti-helix
- Anti-tragus
- Lobule

Microtia

1. Background:
   - Congenital malformation with variable severity of external and middle ear, hearing may be affected

- External ear develops before middle ear; hence, middle ear abnormalities are almost always present
- Male > female
- Rt > Lt
- Unilateral > bilateral
- Association: Only in 5%
  - Branchio-oto-renal syndrome
  - Treacher Collins
  - Goldenhar/hemifacial microsomia (former involves internal organs)
  - Thalidomide
  - Foetal alcohol syndrome
  - Maternal diabetes

2. History:
   - Present as infants or children
3. Examination:
   - Craniofacial microsomia
   - Facial asymmetry and weakness
   - EAC involvement
4. Investigations:
   - Audiology: Bone conduction ABR
   - Renal USS to rule out branchio-oto-renal syndrome
   - Cross-sectional imaging in event of craniofacial microsomia or to assess middle ear/ossicular involvement (high-resolution CT)
5. Management:
   - MDT approach: Dedicated microtia clinic: Genetics, ENT, plastic surgery, audiology, prosthetics
   - Conservative:
     - Purely observational if asymptomatic
     - Hearing rehabilitation:
       - Softband BC device
       - Percutaneous bone conduction implant (age 5, or younger in some children depending on unit). Any device should be sited sufficiently to prevent compromise of reconstruction in the future
       - Depending on ossicular status, middle ear implantation
   - Surgical:
     - For practical purposes, ear is fully developed at 6–7 yrs of age (85% of total size)
     - Costal cartilage growth sufficient by 10 yrs of age, whilst at this age, the patient can also be involved in the decision-making process
     - Intervention timing must be weighed against defect and severity of deformity against age as well as psychosocial aspects
     - Usually two stage with minor revisions

- Procedures:
  - Osseointegrated implants and prosthesis
  - Autologous reconstruction
- Stage 1:
  - Three to four costal segments harvested
  - Lobule rotation
  - Remnant dissection and placement of framework
  - Banking of unused cartilage for stage 2 if required
- Stage 2:
  - 3–4 months later
  - Creation of temporoparietal fascial or postauricular fascial flap
  - Additional defect closed with STSG harvested from posterior scalp
  - Risks: Pneumothorax from cartilage harvesting, cartilage/skin tissue loss, infection, bleeding, numbness, scarring

Weerda Classification:

I: All subunits, but mishappen. Normal EAC
II: Subunits deficient or absent. EAC present but narrow
III: Rudimentary bar. No EAC
IV: Anotia. No EAC

Down Syndrome and ENT Manifestations

1. Background:
   - Trisomy 21
   - Three variants: Mitotic non-disjunction (94%), Robertsonian translocation (3.5%), Mosaicism (2.5%)
   - Association with increased maternal age
   - A ratio of 1:1000 births
   - Life expectancy: Fifth decade
2. History:
   - Cognitive, language and motor delay
   - Ear:
     - Hearing loss (CHL, SNHL and MHL)
   - Nose:
     - Sleep disordered breathing: 60% by 4 yrs of age due to adenoidal hypertrophy, macroglossia and obesity
     - Rhinosinusitis (multi-factorial: Immunodeficiency, crowded nasal profile)

- Throat:
  - Stridor from potential subglottic stenosis
  - Lethargy from hypothyroidism
  - Drooling

3. Examination:
   - Face/head:
     - Flat occiput
     - Flat midface
     - Brachycephaly (coronal synostosis)
     - AA instability (15% of patients), with risk of AA subluxation
   - Eyes:
     - Epicanthic folds
     - Upslanting palpebral fissures
     - Hypertelorism
   - Nose:
     - Hypoplastic nasal bones/low nasal bridge
     - Reduced nasal flow secondary to adenoidal hypertrophy
   - Ears:
     - Small low-set ears with exaggerated helical fold
     - Ear canal stenosis
     - Glue ear (palatal and skull-base anomalies as well as adenoidal hypertrophy)
     - Eustachian tube dysfunction (high risk of cholesteatoma)
   - Throat:
     - OSA (multi-factorial)/pharyngomalacia (hypotonia)
     - Protruding tongue/macroglossia
     - Subglottic stenosis
4. Investigations:
   - Antenatal:
     - USS: Increased nuchal translucency, hypoplastic nasal bones
     - Invasive: Amniocentesis, chorionic villus sampling
     - Triple test: AFP, beta-HCG, oestriol
     - Quadruple test: As above + inhibin A
   - Post-natal:
     - ABR
     - Polysomnography (sleep disordered breathing is a common presentation)
     - Echo: ASD, VSD, PDA
5. Management:
   - MDT approach
   - Genetic counselling
   - Conservative:
     - 3 month observational period
     - Intervention if thresholds of 25–30-dB HL or worse in better ear at 0.5, 1, 2, 4 kHz

    - Hearing aids: First line due to technically challenging nature/anatomy, softband – NICE 2008
  - Medical: No medical intervention
  - Surgical:
    - Grommets considered under exceptional circumstances, as added risk of:
      - Persistent otorrhoea, infection
      - Early extrusion
      - Technicality (anatomical considerations)
    - Adenotonsillectomy: NB risk of atlantoaxial subluxation due to acute dens/facet angle. Minimise hyperextension with head in neutral position. For OSA features

Cleft Lip and Palate

1. Background:
   - Embryology:
     - Three prominences: Maxillary, mandibular and frontonasal
     - Maxilla and mandible form from first pharyngeal arch (week 4)
     - Primary palate: Fusion of frontonasal and maxillary prominences to form lip and alveolus (6 weeks)
     - Secondary palate: Palatal shelves fuse separating oral and nasal cavities (week 9)
     - Failure of fusion of either process will lead to cleft formation
   - A total of 1/1000 lip and 1/2000 palate
   - Asian/native American prevalence
   - Palate (M), lip (F)
   - Syndromes:
     - CHARGE
     - DiGeorge
     - Van der Woude
     - Treacher Collins
     - Goldenhar
   - Risk factors:
     - FH in 25% or older sibling with cleft
     - Teratogens:
       - Thalidomide
       - Retinoids
       - Valproate and carbamazepine
       - Maternal alcohol consumption
       - Smoking
     - Folate deficiency
     - Maternal diabetes

2. History:
   - History of sleep apnoea (PRS)
   - Poor speech development due to palatal and lip defect
   - Poor feeding due to difficult latch and regurgitation, leading to failure to thrive (hence requirement of 10 lb at lip repair)
3. Examination:
   - Examine for other craniofacial abnormalities:
     - Ears: Microtia, pits, tags (Treacher Collins/Goldenhar), CN function (Goldenhar), glue ear (ETD) and cholesteatoma
     - Nose:
       - LL cartilage inferior, with alae retro-displaced
       - Anterior septum and ANS deflected to normal side, along with columella (as attaches to palatine shelf of normal side)
       - Posterior bony septum shifted to cleft side
     - Mandible: Retrognathia (PRS)
     - Lip: Pits in lower lip (Van Der Woude syndrome)
     - Pharynx: Submucous cleft may have muscular (abnormal attachment of TVP) or bony deformity
   - Paediatric assessment: Heart, GU, limb etc.
4. Management:
   - MDT approach: Cleft, ENT surgeons, geneticist, cleft nurse, audiologist, SALT, dentist/orthodontist, psychologist
   - Conservative:
     - Psychological intervention for family as well as child
     - SALT input: Specialised nipples (McGovern, Mead-Johnson), obturator, nursed in upright position
   - Surgical: Remember rule of 10:
     - At birth: Latham appliance: Pins in hard palate, tightened to close palate prior to correction
     - 10 weeks: Lip repair, if 10 lb and Hb 10, tip rhinoplasty, floor repair
     - 10 months: Palate repair ± grommets if failed newborn screening
     - 3–5 yrs: Columella lengthening, tip revision
     - 10 yrs: Dental implants
     - 16 yrs: Definitive rhinoplasty/midfacial advancement
5. Investigations:
   - Sleep studies
   - Yearly audiology

Veau classification: Posterior to anterior

Group I:	Disorder of soft palate only
Group II:	Disorder of soft and hard palate
Group III:	Disorder up to alveolus, with unilateral lip
Groups IV:	Complete bilateral cleft lip and palate

Paediatric Airway Compromise/Stridor

1. Background:
   - Differences in paediatric airway compared to adults:
     - Large occiput
     - Larger tongue
     - Higher larynx (C1–C4, compared to C3–C6)
     - Narrowest portion is subglottis (compared to glottis)
     - Larger omega-shaped epiglottis (immaturity)
2. History:
   - Onset: Progressive (laryngomalacia), sudden (FB)
   - Associated prodrome (epiglottitis, supraglottitis, worsening of pre-existing subglottic stenosis)
   - Level of obstruction: Inspiratory, expiratory, biphasic stridor or stertor
   - Feeding
   - Cyanosis
   - PMH: Previous surgery (cardiac, head and neck), previous intubations/SCBU, haemangiomas (subglottic), immunisations
3. Examination: APLS algorithm:
   - Ensure child is transferred to resuscitation bay or theatre if concerns
   - Prevent distress (avoid BP, oropharyngeal examination or IV access/venepuncture)
     A. Assess for stridor, level, drooling
     B. Tachypnoea, desaturations, cyanosis, tracheal tug, SC/IC/sternal recession, nasal flaring, head bobbing
     C. Tachycardia, dehydration (avoid BP)
     D. GCS (reduced level indicative of fatigue), temperature, assess for cutaneous haemangiomas
4. Investigations:
   - Usually limited, but if stable airway, can undertake soft-tissue XR of neck and chest (steeple sign in croup, thumbprinting in epiglottitis)
5. Management:
   - MDT approach: ENT, anaesthetics, PICU, paediatrics, theatre staff
   - Inform theatres of the need for MLB/age adjusted bronchoscopy kit and tracheostomy set
   - Conservative: Minimise distress, upright posture
   - Medical:
     - High flow oxygen wafted, without tight fit mask
     - Oral antibiotics as per trust guidance
     - Adrenaline nebuliser: 1:1000 made up to 5 mL with saline
     - Dexamethasone PO: 0.15–0.30 mg/kg
   - Surgical:
     - Priority is to secure airway, with anaesthetic team provided with an attempt using anaesthetic laryngoscope and direct view

- If failure, then consider below:
    - Spontaneous breathing with sevoflurane
    - Topical anaesthesia
    - Nasopharyngeal airway
    - Parson's paediatric scope inserted into vallecula
    - View obtained with rigid endoscope
- Once decision made to secure airway, there are two methods:
    - MLB set-up, with ETT sheathed over rigid endoscope, and railroaded once endoscope visualised within trachea
    - Ventilating bronchoscope, bougie and then ETT railroaded, once view obtained within trachea
- If it cannot intubate, cannot ventilate situation:
    - Emergency cricothyrotomy
    - Paediatric tracheostomy

6. Differential diagnoses:
    - Inflammatory: Croup, epiglottitis, supraglottitis, PPS/RPS infection
    - Anatomical: Table 2.1
    - Lesions: Vallecular cyst, papilloma

Site of pathology and characteristic noise

Pharynx:	Stertor
Supraglottis:	Inspiratory stridor
Subglottis:	Biphasic
Trachea:	Expiratory

Table 2.1 Paediatric Stridor

Vascular rings:	**Pulmonary artery sling:**
• Double aortic arch, most common • Bifurcates (ascending aorta) to surround trachea/oesophagus, rejoining descending aorta • Posterior indentation of oesophagus on barium swallow as sandwiches trachea and oesophagus as one	• Lt pulmonary artery arises from the right • Passes between trachea and oesophagus • Right-sided compression of trachea • Anterior compression on barium swallow

(Continued)

Table 2.1 Paediatric Stridor ***(Continued)***

Laryngeal web: • Associated with 22q11 deletion syndrome • CATCH-22 (cardiac, abnormal facies, thymic hypoplasia, cleft, hypocalcaemia/parathyroidism) • Glottic and extend posteriorly due to incomplete re-canalisation of airway • Aphonia, stridor (inspiratory or biphasic), usually when stressed (otherwise asymptomatic) • Laryngofissure + keel • Cohen classification: 20% incremental increase Type 1: 0–35% Type 2: 36–55% Type 3: 56–75% Type 4: >75%	**Tracheo-oesophageal fistula:** • Polyhydramnios on peri-natal USS • Absence of foetal stomach bubble on USS • Congenital or acquired (tracheostomy, intubation, infection) • Gagging at birth, cyanosis, aspiration • Contrast swallow, CXR, echo (cardiac abnormalities), MLB • Corrected with thoracotomy, resection and anastomosis • Gross classification: A–E: NB atresia in A–D A: Oesophageal atresia, no TOF B: Oesophageal atresia, proximal TOF C: Oesophageal atresia, distal TOF D: Oesophageal atresia, bilateral TOF E: TOF (no atresia)

Laryngeal cleft:
• Failure of oesophagotracheal ridges to fuse
• Aspiration risk
• Types 1–3 repaired endoscopically, 4 with laryngofissure
• Benjamin-Inglis classification:
Type 1: To vocal cords
Type 2: Partial cricoid
Type 3: Through posterior cricoid/ cervical trachea
Type 4: Involvement of thoracic trachea
	Vocal cord paralysis:
	• Unilateral > bilateral
	• Causes:
	  • Congenital: Chiari malformation
	  • Idiopathic
	  • Iatrogenic: Birth trauma, surgery (thoracic/mediastinal, head & neck)
	  • Infection: Encephalitis, syphilis, polio
	  • Hydrocephalus
	• MRI (Chiari malformation) & MLB
	• Most usually resolve within 6–12 months
	• Tracheostomy to secure airway with periodic MLB (approx. 50% of bilateral VC palsies)

Tracheomalacia: • Most common congenital anomaly of trachea • Primary: Prematurity (improves as cartilage stiffens), as is trachea-oesophageal fistula • Secondary: Due to prolonged intubation, tracheostomy, extrinsic compression (CT, MRI)	

Laryngomalacia

1. Background:
   - Most common cause of paediatric stridor. Onset within first 2 weeks of life, worsening at 6/12, resolution by 2 yrs
   - Prevalence of 50%
   - Male > female
   - Aetiology:
     - Neurological
     - Immature cartilage
     - Mucosal oedema secondary to GORD or trauma on collapse
   - Not associated with prematurity, hence refutes immature cartilage theory
   - Exacerbated by GORD, and seen in 50% of population
   - If left untreated, may lead to failure to thrive, apnoea, cyanosis, CCF/cor pulmonale, pectus excavatum
2. History:
   - History of presenting complaint:
     - Timing/onset:
       - Immediate = Subglottic stenosis (congenital), web, VF palsy (Arnold-Chiari malformation)
       - Weeks to months = Laryngomalacia
       - Year = Papilloma
     - Positioning (worse supine = laryngomalacia)
     - Crying (improves pyriform aperture stenosis and choanal atresia, worsens laryngomalacia)
     - Issues with feeding (choanal atresia, pyriform aperture stenosis, trachea-oesophageal fistula)
     - Poor weight gain/failure to thrive (airway pathology and energy expenditure due to difficulties co-ordinating feeds)
     - Cyanosis
     - GORD symptoms (exacerbates subglottic stenosis and laryngomalacia)
     - Assess for chest infections/aspiration
   - PMH:
     - Birthing history: Premature (trachea-oesophageal fistula), instrumentation delivery (VF palsy)
     - Previous surgery/intubations (subglottic stenosis, VF palsy)
     - Cardiac history, with previous surgery (cyanosis, and suspected VF palsy)
3. Examination:
   - NB: ABCDE assessment, focusing particularly on A and B
   - Evaluate weight: If dropping centiles, evidence of moderate/severe disease
   - Evaluation of voice and stridor

   - Signs of increased work of breathing: Cyanosis (desaturation), tachypnoea, tracheal tug, IC/SC/sternal recession
   - FNE: Assess degree of laryngomalacia and VF movement
4. Investigations:
   - USS vocal cords if suspected VF palsy
5. Management:
   - Conservative: In 70% of individuals:
     - Postural changes with feeds
     - Thickened feeds
   - Medical:
     - NG feeding in extreme cases of failure to thrive, which may improve symptoms
     - PPI therapy for GORD ± paediatric Gaviscon
   - Surgical:
     - MLB: Diagnosis of secondary airway lesions: High as 30%, but accepted figure is 10%
       - Findings:
         - Long tubular, retro-displaced epiglottis (omega-shaped)
         - Anterior collapse of arytenoids
         - Tight aryepiglottic folds
         - Indrawing of aryepiglottic folds
       - Technique:
         - If supraglottic collapse, mount Lindholm scope with microscope
         - Division of aryepiglottic folds and trimming of excess mucosa (cold steel, CO_2 laser or microdebrider)
       - Risks: GA, bleeding, worsening in airway symptoms, orodental trauma, aspiration, supraglottic stenosis (from excess reduction in posterior commissure)

Subglottic Stenosis

1. Background:
   - Normal = 7 mm
     - <4 mm in newborn or <3.5 mm in premature child is diagnostic of SGS
2. History:
   - Recurrent croup in otherwise well child
   - Failed extubation (usually two permitted in most children), but must be taken in context (multiple morbidities, lung function as other causes of failure)
   - PMH: SCBU stay, previous intubations and duration

3. Examination:
   - NB: ABCDE assessment, focusing particularly on A and B
   - Evaluate weight: If dropping centiles, evidence of moderate/severe disease
   - Evaluation of voice and stridor
   - Signs of increased work of breathing: Cyanosis (desaturation), tachypnoea, tracheal tug, IC/SC/sternal recession
   - FNE
4. Management:
   - Conservative:
     - Mainly for grade 1 subglottic stenosis
     - Medical:
       - Antibiotics as per trust guidance, if bacterial infection suspected
       - Dexamethasone (0.15–0.30 mg/kg)
       - Adrenaline nebuliser (1 mg/mL of 1:1000 made to 5 mL or neat)
     - Surgical:
       - MLB ± incision (dependent on site/length/maturity of stenosis) + dilatation ± Mitomycin C injection (DNA cross linker formed from streptomycin bacteria, which inhibits fibroblast proliferation and is deemed a chemotherapeutic agent)
       - Laser use controversial
       - LTR: Cricoid split and grafting: Doubling the radius will increase flow 16 folds
         - Best benefit quoted in children 10 kg and above
         - Reconstruction with cartilage, usually required for grade 3 and above
         - Anterior is undertaken as an open approach due to presence of isthmus and likelihood of bleeding
         - Posterior split can be undertaken endoscopically
         - Done as single or double stage (second stage is decannulating tracheostomy)
         - Single stage means decannulating at same time and can be done for A and P or both grafts
         - Second stage is reserved for children with multiple co-morbidities (cardiorespiratory), and unlikely to be able to extubate, as well as for AP grafting
         - Graft is usually costal or thyroid ala
         - Stented and intubated for 1/52 if single stage
         - 50% decannulation success rate
       - Cricotracheal resection (starting below vocal folds) + anastomosis:
         - Usually single stage
         - For grade III and IV (only option for grade IV)
         - Involves resection of cricoid and thyrotracheal closure
         - 90% decannulation success rate

- Slide tracheoplasty: For long segmental tracheal stenosis
  - For long stenotic segment involving trachea
  - Lower lip of tracheal segment kept, which is placed over posterior surface of cricoid and framework sutured
  - Anterior segment of cricoid resected
  - Soft tissue (stenotic segment) removed from posterior aspect of cricoid + resurfaced with drill

Congenital causes: Elliptical, failure to re-canalise (small diameter cricoid), prematurity, can be membranous, cartilaginous or mixed, cartilaginous non-responsive to dilatation.

Acquired causes: Circumferential trauma, GORD, high tracheostomy, infections, intubations (Cole's tube), thin and friable, hence easier to dilate, segment longer and thicker when more established.

Cotton-Meyer grading:

I: 0–50% endoscopic treatment
II: 51–70% endoscopic treatment
III: 71–99% resting stridor
IV: 100%

Thyroglossal Duct Cyst

1. Background:
   - Most common midline neck cyst
   - Failure of thyroglossal duct to obliterate (formed from tract as thyroid descends from tuberculum impar to midline)
   - Midline (90%) > left (9%) > right (1%)
   - 75% infra-hyoid
   - The TGDC is the only thyroid tissue present in 1% of cases. Can consider scintigraphy if there are concerns regarding functional thyroid tissue
   - Lined by respiratory and squamous epithelium
   - Can be dormant and present following trauma
   - Low risk of papillary ca (95%) or SCC (5%) – literature <1–3%
2. History:
   - Length of lump
   - Increase in size
   - Infections
   - Extrinsic compression (dysphagia, dysphonia, dyspnoea)
   - PMH: Congenital anomalies
   - FH: Thyroid disease

3. Examination:
   - Full head and neck examination focusing on lesion:
     - Skin changes
     - Tenderness
     - Mobility with swallowing or tongue protrusion
   - Evaluation of other neck lumps
   - Assessment for congenital abnormalities in head and neck
4. Investigations:
   - USS in initial instance to assess lesion as well as presence of normal thyroid gland
   - Scintigraphy to localise functional thyroid tissue
   - TFT may be considered
5. Management:
   - Conservative: Can be offered to parents in asymptomatic child, but always provide risk of malignancy
   - Medical: Antibiotics during acute inflammation ± aspiration
   - Surgical: Modified Sistrunk procedure:
     - Prepped as per thyroidectomy
     - Local anaesthetic
     - Skin crease if healthy skin, or elliptical incision, including scarred tissue or fistula
     - Medial aspect of strap muscles dissected (this along with isthmus dissection would be described as an extended Sistrunk procedure)
     - Middle 1/3 of hyoid excised
     - Triangular buff of tissue from hyoid to tongue base excised with bimanual palpation of tongue base
     - Drain insertion (Concertina)
     - Straps and platysma closed
     - Subcuticular closure with Monocryl
   - Surgical options: Cyst excision alone (high recurrence rate) ± hyoid ± core of tongue-base tissue ± en-bloc extended soft-tissue dissection
     - If multiple recurrences, consider panendoscopy to rule out tongue-base thyroglossal duct cyst
   - If papillary carcinoma seen, treatment is total thyroidectomy with RAI
6. Differential diagnoses:
   - Thyroid nodule (adenoma or carcinoma)
   - Midline dermoid
   - Lipoma
   - Vascular malformation
   - Ranula
   - Reactive lymphadenopathy

Lingual thyroid:

- 70% of patients are hypothyroid at presentation
- Malignant transformation rare
- Present with symptoms of airway lesion: Assess for red flags
- Midline base of tongue swelling on FNE
- Investigations: TFTs, USS (assess for normal thyroid), CT, FNAC, scintigraphy
- May require lip-split procedure to excise/TORS, reduction with coblation, RAI ablation
- Resected thyroid may be re-implanted if only functioning tissue

Vascular Anomalies (Haemangiomas)

1. Background:
   - Categorised as congenital (vascular malformations) or acquired (haemangiomas of infancy, malignancy beyond infancy)
   - A benign vascular tumour, of endothelial origin
   - Congenital vs infantile
   - Glut-1 overexpression ONLY seen in infantile
   - Congenital haemangiomas can either involute within a year or remain as it is
   - 50% regress by 5 yrs, 70% by 7 yrs, 80% by 9 yrs
   - Superficial (capillary), deep (cavernous), compound (mixed)
   - Parotid most common benign lesion in children
   - 50% of subglottic lesions will have cutaneous lesions, but only 1% of cutaneous lesions will have subglottic haemangioma
   - Beard distribution associated with higher incidence of subglottic haemangiomas
   - PHACES syndrome:
     - P(osterior fossa) anomalies
     - H(aemangiomas)
     - A(rterial) anomalies
     - C(ardiac) anomalies
     - E(ye) anomalies
     - Sternal pit
     - Propranolol can cause stroke in PHACES, hence exclude before initiating (MRA)
2. History:
   - Age of onset, presence of any herald patches at birth to suggest congenital
   - Location
   - Progression in size

- Airway symptoms in neck
- Pain/ulceration/skin changes
- Location (eye associated with intracranial and beard with subglottic involvement)
- PMH: Any other concerns such as cardiac anomalies, visual defects to suggest PHACES

3. Examination:
   - Assessment of lesion location, size, pain, ulceration/skin changes, bruit/thrill
   - Examination for other cutaneous lesions in the head and neck or torso
   - Assessment for stridor (subglottic) ± FNE if possible
4. Investigations:
   - FBC: Platelet consumption (Kasabach-Merritt syndrome)
     - Thrombocytopaenia associated with haemangiothelioma
     - Caused by platelet trapping within tumour
   - USS/Doppler to quantify if low or high flow
   - CV examination, ECG, Echo prior to initiation of propranolol (rule out high output CCF)
   - MRI head to rule out posterior fossa lesions (PHACES) or if lesions in upper half of face
   - MLB for suspected cases
5. Management:
   - Conservative: For asymptomatic lesions
   - Medical:
     - Steroids (especially if propranolol contraindicated/non-responder)
     - Propranolol (check for hypoglycaemia): 1 mg/kg three divided doses, increased to 2 mg/kg. Up to 3 mg/kg for minimum 12 months
       - Proposed mechanism: Downregulates VEGF
       - Vasoconstriction causes softening of haemangioma
     - Vincristine or interferon (if >12/12)
   - Surgical:
     - Pulsed-dye laser
     - Excision
     - For subglottic haemangioma:
       - MLB + microdebrider
       - Laryngofissure and excision for large circumferential lesions

Stages:

Proliferative (<12 months):	Endothelial cell hyperplasia, increased mitosis
Involuting:	50% regress by 5 yrs, 70% by 7 yrs, fibrosis, reduced cellularity
Involuted:	Soft mass, excess skin, fibrofatty tissue

Vascular Anomalies (Vascular Malformations)

1. Background:
   - Present at birth, and do NOT regress unlike haemangiomas
   - Progresses in size with child
     - Can cause DIC and mortality
   - Based on flow:
     - High flow: AVM
       - Slow growth followed by rapid growth in second/third decade (puberty/trauma)
     - Low flow:
       - Lymphatic:
         - Macrocystic: >1 cyst, thick walled and easier to resect, at least 2 cm large
         - Microcystic: <2 cm, thin walls, invade tissues, i.e. tongue muscles, and are usually suprahyoid
         - Mixed: Lymphangioma/cystic hygroma
       - Capillary:
         - Port wine stain
         - If on face and thigh – Klippel-Trenaunay
         - Sturge-Weber: Port-wine stain over CNV distribution with epilepsy (leptomeningeal extension)
       - Venous:
         - Rapid growth during with age due to hormonal changes
         - Can get thrombosis
2. History:
   - Age of onset
   - Location
   - Progression in size
   - Airway symptoms in neck
   - Pain/ulceration/skin changes
   - Location (eye associated with intracranial and beard with subglottic involvement)
   - PMH: Any other concerns such as cardiac anomalies, visual defects to suggest PHACES
3. Examination:
   - Assessment of lesion location, size, pain, ulceration/skin changes, bruit/thrill
   - Examination for other cutaneous lesions in the head and neck or torso
   - Assessment for stridor (subglottic) ± FNE if possible
4. Investigations:
   - High flow:
     - Doppler, MRA/CTA

- Lymphatic:
  - MRI

5. Management:
   - High flow:
     - Embolisation
     - Rarely surgical
   - Low flow:
     - Lymphatic:
       - Surgical excision for macrocystic (subtotal for suprahyoid to preserve critical structures)
       - Sclerotherapy for macrocystic
       - Coblation for microcystic disease on tongue, oral cavity except floor of mouth
     - Capillary:
       - Pulsed-dye laser
     - Venous:
       - Surgery if well defined
       - Pulsed-dye laser
       - Sclerotherapy (OK-432, Bleomycin)

Schobinger classification for AVM

I:	Quiescent stage
II:	Expansion (bruit, thrill, throbbing)
III:	Destruction (bleeding, ulcers)
IV:	High-output CCF

Lymphatic malformation classification:

Stage I:	Unilateral, infrahyoid
Stage II:	Unilateral, suprahyoid
Stage III:	Unilateral, infra- and suprahyoid
Stage IV:	Bilateral, infrahyoid
Stage V:	Bilateral, infra- and suprahyoid

Obstructive Sleep Apnoea (Paediatric)

1. Background:
   - AHI:

Normal	0
Mild:	1–5
Moderate:	5–10
Severe:	>10

- Risk factors: Age (2–6), craniofacial abnormalities, neuromuscular disorders, obesity, mucopolysaccharidoses

2. History:
   - Witnessed apnoea or snoring (NB OSA is a spectrum)
   - Nocturnal enuresis
   - Sweating
   - Hyperactivity/restlessness
   - Poor concentration/erratic behaviour/school concerns
   - Weight loss
   - Woken by parents in the morning for nursery/school
   - PMH:
     - Down's syndrome
     - Neurological disease (cerebral palsy)
     - Craniofacial abnormalities (Apert's, Crouzon's, Pfeiffer's syndromes)
3. Examination:
   - Oropharyngeal examination: Tonsillar hypertrophy
   - Anterior rhinoscopy/FNE: Adenoidal hypertrophy
4. Investigations:
   - Clinical examination with cold spatula test, in children where examination with FNE is difficult
   - Indications for polysomnography (local policies):
     - <5 kg/2 yrs if referring to tertiary centre
     - Unclear diagnosis
     - Syndromic children: Down's, craniofacial abnormalities
     - Neuromuscular disorders
     - Significant co-morbidities (CHD, CLD), where benefits must outweigh risk
     - Continued OSA symptoms post adenotonsillectomy
   - Polysomnography: EEG, electro-oculography (assess stage of sleeping), nasal/oral flow, chest/abdominal expansion, HR, sats, CO_2 and EMG (for parasomnias). Will not show level of obstruction
   - Domiciliary sleep study: Portable device. Will not measure EEG, EOG, EMG or CO_2
5. Management:
   - Conservative/lifestyle: Observational period, as most cases resolve by 8 yrs of age
   - Medical: CPAP
   - Surgery:
     - Adenotonsillectomy:
       - ■ Cold steel ± suction diathermy combination
       - ■ Coblation tonsillotomy:
         - o Use of RF energy passed through saline
         - o Formation of a plasma field

      - o Lower energy of 40–70 degrees
      - o Breaks intracellular bonds in tissue
      - o 2% regrowth rate of tissue requiring further surgery
      - o Low risk:
        - Lower bleeding risk
        - Lower temperature compared to electrocautery
        - Capsule intact leading to less post-operative pain and quicker recovery
  - Process if symptoms do not subside:
    - Repeat sleep studies
    - Assess for regrowth/remnants/alternative nasal pathology
    - Consider referring to respiratory for CPAP
  - Indications for referral to specialist centre:
    - <2 yrs or <15 kg
    - Neuromuscular disorders
    - Severe OSA
    - Co-morbidities, i.e. obesity (Prader-Willi) or craniofacial abnormalities

Paediatric Hearing Loss

1. Background:
   - Incidence of congenital hearing loss is 1:1000
   - Genetic: 50% of cases
     - A total of 1/3 syndromic (Table 2.2):
       - ■ Chromosomal: Down, Patau, Turner's syndrome
       - ■ Autosomal dominant hearing loss: Post-lingual, and progressive
         - o WANT CBS: Waardenburg, Apert, NF, Treacher Collins, Crouzon, Branchio-oto-renal syndromes, Stickler
       - ■ Autosomal recessive hearing loss: Pre-lingual, and profound (more severe)
         - o PURJ: Pendred, Usher, Refsum, Jervell-Lange-Niellson
       - ■ X-linked: Alport syndrome
     - A total of 2/3 non-syndromic: Most common:
       - ■ Autosomal recessive non-syndromic hearing loss = connexin-26 (GJB2 gene mutation)
       - ■ Connexin-26, gap junction protein that permits intra-cellular ion transport in basement membrane and stria vascularis
   - Acquired:
     - Maternal: Alcoholism, DM
     - Prematurity (ex SCBU) + low APGAR score at birth
     - Inflammatory:

Table 2.2 Syndromes in ENT

Autosomal Dominant: WANT-CBS	*Autosomal Recessive: PURJG*
Waardenburg syndrome: • SNHL: Poor melanocyte differentiation in stria vascularis • Pigmentation abnormalities (heterochromia iridis, patchy skin and white forelock) • Hypertelorism • Type 1 and 2: Hearing loss, unibrow and forelock in both • Dystopia canthorum only present in type 1 (inner canthus displacement), with less severe hearing loss • Hirschsprung's disease in type 4	**Pendred syndrome:** • Genetics: SLC26A4 • Pendrin: Chloride as well as Iodide transport • Multi-nodular goitre, clinically euthyroid, although 50% hypothyroid • +ve Perchlorate test (increased iodine release with Perchlorate) • Enlarged vestibular aqueduct or Mondini defect • SNHL > CHL
Apert syndrome (acrocephalosyndactyly): • FGFR2 mutation • Lambdoid and coronal suture • Brachycephaly most common • SNHL and CHL (stapes fixation) • Low nasal bridge • Syndactyly/webbing of hands or feet • Hypertelorism • Proptosis	**Usher syndrome:** • Most common cause of HL and blindness • Retinitis pigmentosa • Cataracts • Type 1: Vestibular dysfunction and profound HL • Type 2: Moderate HL (most common) • Type 3 is a milder phenotype of type 1
Treacher Collins syndrome: • Mandibulofacial dysostosis • TCOF1 mutation (80%) or POLR1C mutation autosomal dominant, POLR1 mutation autosomal recessive • Hypoplasia of maxilla, zygoma, Malar flattening • Micrognathia • Cleft palate • Coloboma and downslanted palpebral fissures • Microtia and Middle ear abnormalities. CHL • Normal intelligence	**Refsum disease:** • Overaccumulation of phytanic acid in cells/tissues • Due to PHYH mutations • Retinitis pigmentosa • Ataxia • Peripheral weakness

(Continued)

Table 2.2 Syndromes in ENT ***(Continued)***

Autosomal Dominant: WANT-CBS	*Autosomal Recessive: PURJG*
Crouzon syndrome (craniofacial dysostosis): • FGFR2 mutation • CHL > SNHL • Coronal and sagittal suture • Brachycephaly • Midface hypoplasia • Hypertelorism and proptosis • Parrot beak nose • Proptosis • Cleft lip/palate Normal intelligence	**Jervell-Lange-Nielsen syndrome:** • Prolonged QT interval, leading to sudden death • Long arm chromosome 11 (Jerve11) • Mutation affecting potassium channel gene *KCNQ1* • Treatment with beta blockers/ defib
Branchio-oto-renal syndrome: • EYA1, SIX1, SIX5 mutations • Branchial arch anomalies (external ear, pits, sinuses) • Renal dysplasia or hypoplasia • Medially displaced carotid artery • Mixed, conductive (malformed ears or pits) or SNHL	**Goldenhar syndrome:** • First and second arch anomalies • External ear (tags, atresia, microtia, anotia (CHL), SSC, oval window (SNHL) • Semicircular canal aplasia association • Hemifacial microsomia (mandible, soft palate, orbit, muscles)

Stickler syndrome:
• COL2A1 mutation. Four types. No ocular abnormalities in three
• SNHL
• Retinal detachment, cataracts (collagen defect)
• Tall and thin (stick-ler), with hypermobility
• Pierre-robin sequence: Retrognathia, glossoptosis and airway obstruction:
  • Associated with syndrome in 80% of cases
  • Conditions associated: S(tickler), T(reacher-Collins), A(lcohol, foetal syndrome), B(eckwith-Wiedeman), M(obius), D(i George) syndromes	

(Continued)

Table 2.2 Syndromes in ENT *(Continued)*

Autosomal Dominant: WANT-CBS	*Autosomal Recessive: PURJG*
22q11 deletion syndrome: • DiGeorge's syndrome • Chromosome 22 deletion (22q11.2) • Associated with CHARGE (cleft) • Medial deviation of ICA. VPI repair following FNE • CATCH-22: C(ardiac abnormalities), A(bnormal facies), T(hymic hypoplasia), C(left palate), H(ypoparathyroidism/ hypocalcaemia)	
Pfeiffer syndrome: • Similar presentation to Apert syndrome • Turribrachycephaly • Three types, with two and three being severe with poor prognosis • FGFR1 and FGFR2 mutations • Normal intelligence Syndactyly and hallux valgus	**X linked:** **Alport syndrome:** • Type 4 collagen mutation, COL4A5 • Basement membrane defect • Progressive renal disease: Microscopic and macroscopic haematuria & ESRF • SNHL, present in adolescence - EVA Ophthalmic signs: Retinal flecks
Achondroplasia • Dwarfism • FGFR3 Gene, autosomal dominant • Macrocephaly • Anteverted nares, depressed nasal bridge, frontal bossing, short nasal bridge • Deafness, middle ear abnormalities • OSA • Normal Intelligence • Small fingers, limited range of motion of elbows, bowing of legs, lumbar hyperlordosis, knee hypermobility	

      - TORCH: Toxoplasmosis, Other (syphilis, varicella), Rubella, CMV, Herpes Simplex
      - Meningitis: High risk of cochlear ossification hence fast track for CI
    - Trauma
    - Ototoxicity
    - Jaundice/hyperbilirubinaemia
  - Newborn hearing screening: Set-up in 2005: two pathways. Done within 4 weeks
    - SCBU/NICU pathway (IF >48 hrs): 10× higher risk of hearing loss
      - AOAE + ABR (one attempt)
      - Any failure, gets referred to audiology
    - Well baby pathway:
      - AOAE (two attempts), then ABR if fail again, if pass, discharge
      - High risk or failures always get referred to audiology (craniofacial abnormalities, ototoxicity, TORCH, FH, failed OAE)
    - Not done on premature children <34 weeks as auditory cortex not developed
  - Otoacoustic emissions: Assesses cochlear function, hence normal in auditory neuropathy. Absent in OME
    - Sound generated by outer hair cells (organ of Corti) in response to auditory stimuli (click = wide, tone = narrow)
      - Evoked occur after stimuli: Two used cover low and high frequencies
        - o Transient (TEOAE): Used in neonatal screening. Response at multiple frequencies up to 4 kHz
        - o Distortion product (DPOAE): Two simultaneous pure tones at two frequencies (stimulates more of basilar membrane)
        - o Measures at higher frequencies (1–8 kHz) so used for NIHL and ototoxicity

2. History:
   - Age and onset of symptoms (if newborn then likely picked up on neonatal screening)
   - Speech development for age and school progression
   - History of infections (OME, AOM)
   - PMH: Gestation, delivery Hx, Neonatal screening, TORCH infections, meningitis, HDU/ITU admission, ventilation
   - DH: Ototoxic medications
   - FH: Of early onset hearing loss
3. Examination:
   - Ear/auricle
   - Syndromic features
   - Otoscopy

4. Investigations:
   - Genetic testing (connexin 26, pendrin)
   - MRI IAM (CN 7, 8 and labyrinth) or CT (bony anatomy)
   - Renal USS (BORS)
   - ECG (Jervell-Lange-Nielson syndrome)
   - Blood tests: FBC, TFTs (Pendred), urinalysis (Alport syndrome), serology for CMV and syphilis, IgM (toxoplasma and rubella)
   - Ophthalmology referral
5. Management:
   - MDT approach
   - Counselling (genetic)
   - Trial of hearing aids early
   - Consider for cochlear implantation

Paediatric hearing tests

- 0–6 M: AOAE
- 6M–3 yrs: VRA (headphones or speakers, turns to auditory signal with reward for visual stimulus), ±OAE, ±ABR
- 2–5 yrs: CPA (conditioned play audiometry): Performs task in response to noise
- 5+yrs: PTA

TORCH:

T-oxoplasmosis
O-ther, syphilis, VZ
R-ubella
C-ytomegalovirus
H-erpes, HSV

Branchial Anomalies

1. Introduction:
   - Cysts (no opening)
   - Sinus (single opening)
   - Fistula occurs when there is a connection between pouch and arch
   - Clefts 2–4 have one common opening, hence cannot elicit site based on opening
   - Classifications:
     - Work: Type I (ectoderm), type II (ectoderm and mesoderm)
     - Olsen: Type I (cyst), type II (sinus), type III (fistula)

- Types:
  - First cleft (2%):
    - Type 1:
      - Ectodermal in origin
      - Pre-auricular/tragal ending in mesotympanum
      - Parallel to EAC
      - Superficial to CN VII (not related directly)
    - Type 2:
      - Ectodermal and mesodermal in origin
      - Starts at angle of mandible
      - May be found within substance of parotid
      - Intimately related to facial nerve branches
      - Terminating within EAC
  - Second cleft (90%):
    - Second arch merges with epicardial ridge, ectoderm is trapped forming inclusion cysts form ± sinus or tract
    - Abnormality anterior to SCM, upper border
    - Stratified squamous lining, lymphoid tissue in walls and cholesterol crystals in fluid
    - Starts in anterior neck, along carotid sheath, between ICA and ECA, superficial to CN IX and XII
    - Opens into middle constrictors or tonsillar fossa
  - Third and Fourth cleft (8%):
    - 90% occur on Lt side
    - Passes behind internal carotid artery, between hypoglossal and glossopharyngeal nerves
    - Open into piriform sinus, piercing thyrohyoid membrane
    - Present as suppurative thyroiditis

2. History:
   - Fluctuating mass usually associated with URTI or
   - Discharging sinus/fistula
   - In adult always elicit red flags: Dysphagia, dysphonia, dyspnoea, otalgia + smoking/drinking history as cyst indistinguishable from necrotic node
3. Examination:
   - Full head and neck examination:
     - Oropharynx (second arch anomaly or oropharyngeal site of nodal disease)
     - Location and position of sinus, fistula or cyst (mobility, border, size) as well as other potentially palpable nodes
     - FNE (site of potential nodal disease as well as evaluation of PF for third/fourth arch anomalies)
   - Ear examination: Type I/II anomaly

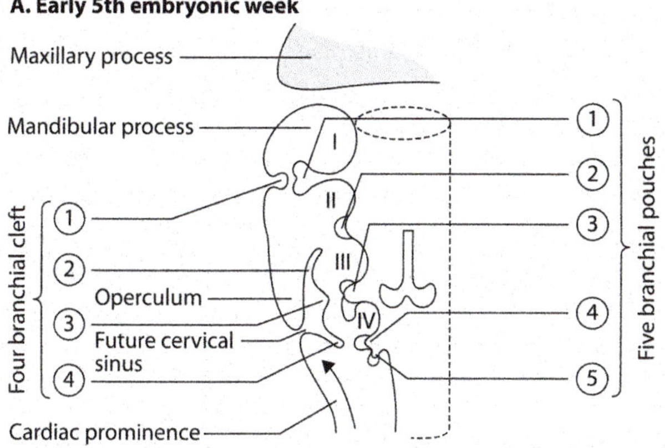

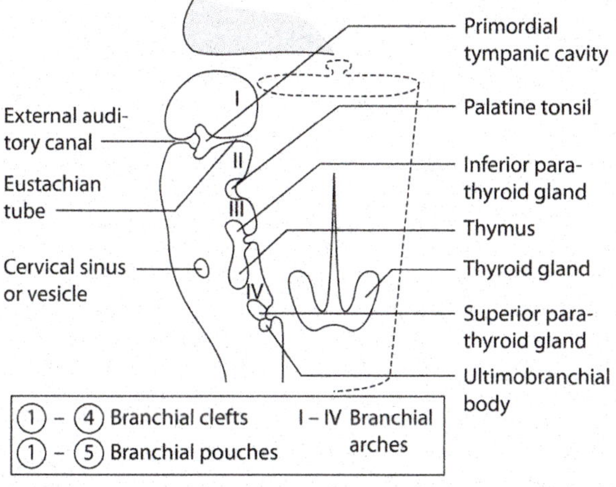

Figure 2.1 Branchial arches, clefts and pouches.

4. Investigations:
   - Genetics (Branchio-oto-renal syndrome)
     - Renal USS
   - MRI: For first cleft anomalies to assess relation to CN VII
   - Fistulogram rarely undertaken
   - Barium swallow for third/fourth cleft anomalies
5. Management:
   - Conservative: If minimal symptoms
   - Medical: For infective episodes
   - Surgical:
     - Aspiration in event of acute infection/abscess to minimise scar tissue
     - First cleft: Excision using facial nerve monitor and parotid approach

- Second cleft:
  - Elliptical incision ± stepladder approach for older children
  - Close dissection of tract using lacrimal probe (no branches)
  - Ligation when entering pharynx
  - Closure in layers
  - Morbidity has minimised excision of ipsilateral tonsil
- Third cleft:
  - Either panendoscopy with diathermy of fistula (common practice) or
  - Radical excision, ±hemithyroidectomy

Paediatric Tracheostomy

1. Background:
   - All forms provided with introducer
   - Most will be single lumen to maximise internal diameter for ventilation
   - Flanges can be straight or V-shaped
   - Categories:
     - Paediatric: Longer inner cannula length. 2.5–6.5 mm diameter
     - Neonatal: Shorter inner cannula length
   - Cuff status:
     - Cuffed: Ventilation and airway protection
     - Uncuffed: Facilitate weaning and vocalisation
   - Brand:
     - Bivona:
       - Silicone (hydrophobic)
       - Metal content, hence caution with MRI
       - Can be cuffed or uncuffed
       - Cuff properties:
         - Fome-cuff: Self-expanding
         - Tight-to-shaft: High pressure, low volume water cuff with tight fit once deflated. Aids insertion. Easier to vocalise than other deflated cuffs which occupy lumen
       - Flange properties:
         - Hyperflex: Variable internal cannula length
         - Flextend: Provides additional external tube length for children with increased neck circumference/AP distance. Resulting in less irritation to skin/excoriation. Aids suctioning and ventilation attachment
     - Shiley:
       - Available in neonatal, standard and long

        - o Only manufacturer of size 5.0–6.5
        - o Aids in bypassing obstructive pathology (cystic hygromas)
        - o Plastic material and disposable after 1/52 use
        - o V-shaped flange may aid better fit dependent on age, with straight-flanges preferred in neonates
        - o Can be cuffed or uncuffed
    - Tracoe twist:
        - ■ Adolescent use
        - ■ Children with less head control
        - ■ Inner tube present, requiring minimal 4-hrs changes/cleaning

2. Paediatric tracheostomy procedure:
    - Positioning: Shoulder roll for neck extension
    - Infiltration of skin with Lignospan
    - Horizontal or vertical incision midway between cricoid cartilage and suprasternal notch
    - Hypodermal fat excised to reveal strap muscles
    - Midline strap division
    - Division of thyroid isthmus with bipolar to enable visualisation of trachea
    - 3.0 Prolene stay sutures either side of incision line
    - Vertical incision between second and fourth tracheal rings (NB no window created)
    - 4 × 3.0 Vicryl stoma maturation sutures. May have to close stay sutures to reduce leak intermittently to allow for oxygenation
    - Anaesthetic colleagues to withdraw ET above stoma but not fully out of airway so ET can be replaced easily, if tracheostomy is unable to be inserted
    - Tracheostomy inserted using introducer
    - Introducer removed and tracheostomy tube is connected to anaesthetic circuit. Assess for end-tidal $CO2$ and chest wall movement. When satisfactory remove ET
    - Tracheostomy tube secured with twill ties
    - CXR in recovery/post-operative ward (likely intensive care)
    - Complications:
        - Early: Haemorrhage, surgical emphysema, pneumomediastinum, pneumothorax, decannulation, mucous plugging
        - Late: Granulation (suprastomal or stomal), haemorrhage, decannulation/false passage, mucous plugging, tracheomalacia, tracheocutaneous fistula, dysphagia, death
    - Decannulation protocol:
        - Original airway issue resolved. Safe upper airway
        - No oxygen requirement
        - Recent MLB to assess airway

- Follow local protocol (e.g.):
    - Day 1: Admit and downsize to size 3.0
    - Day 2: Cap in day time and into night if tolerated
    - Day 3: Remove tracheostomy and dress. Observe in ward
    - Day 4: Able to leave ward but stay in hospital
    - Day 5: Home

Chapter 3

Otology

Jameel Muzaffar, Chloe Swords, Adnan Darr, Karan Jolly, Manohar Bance and Sanjiv Bhimrao

Contents

DOI: 10.1201/9781003247098-3

Common Otology Prescriptions, Ingredients and Procedure

Gentisone:	Gentamicin 0.3% + Hydrocortisone acetate 1%
Locortan vioform:	Clioquinol 1% (anti-fungal) + Flumetasone pivalate 0.02%
Otomize:	Neomycin sulfate 0.5% + Dexamethasone 0.1% + Glacial acetic acid 2%
Otosporin:	Polymyxin B 10,000 U/mL + Neomycin 3400 U/mL + Hydrocortisone 1%
Sofradex:	Framycetin sulfate 0.5% + G<u>ra</u>micidin 0.005% + <u>De</u>xamethasone 0.05%
Canesten:	Clotrimazole 1%
Synalar:	Fluocinolone acetonide 0.025% + Neomycin 0.35%, Polymyxin B 10,000 U/mL

Steroid potency:

Mild:	Hydrocortisone 1%
Moderate:	Betamethasone valerate 0.025%, Clobetasone butyrate 0.05% (Eumovate)
Potent:	Bethamethasone valerate 0.1% (Betnovate), Hydrocortisone butyrate 0.1%, Fluocinolone acetonide 0.025%
Very potent:	Clobetasol propionate 0.05% (Dermovate)

Intratympanic steroid injection:

Equipment:	Speculum, binocular microscope, 25-ga spinal needle, 1 mL syringe
Local anaesthetic:	Varies, cotton wool soaked with EMLA (Eutectic Mixture of Local Anaesthetics) 5% or 70% phenol, 10% xylocaine spray 30 min, subcutaneous injection
Steroid:	Methylprednisolone 30–62.5 mg/mL (depo-medrone® 40 mg/mL (1 mL in each vial)) OR dexamethasone 3.3 mg/mL (equivalent to 4 mg/mL dexamethasone phosphate) OR triamcinolone Ensure at body temperature to prevent caloric reaction, preservation free
Procedure:	0.4–0.8 mL into anteroinferior TM, consider secondary perforation to relieve pressure or grommet if regular intratympanic administration required

Patient advice: No yawning, swallowing or speaking for 20–30 min
Complications: Transient dizziness, burning sensation, ear fullness, headache, perforation, tinnitus, infection, hearing loss, tongue numbness

Ototoxicity

1. Background:
   - Damage to both cochlea and vestibular system
   - High frequencies in initial instance due to basal turn of cochlea being affected initially, followed by apex
2. History:
   - Onset/timing (usually abrupt)
   - Unilateral vs bilateral
   - Associated tinnitus/vertigo/discharge
   - PMH: Previous surgery, previous hearing loss, other causes of hearing level (HL) (idiopathic, iatrogenic, traumatic, infective, neoplastic), renal disease (impaired excretion)
   - DH: Any of above medications initiated prior to onset (see Table 3.1)
   - FH: Aminoglycoside sensitivity

Table 3.1 Common Ototoxic Medications

Antibiotics
• Aminoglycosides: Damage OHCs and IHCs
  • Streptomycin, Gentamicin, Neomycin, Kanamycin, Amikacin, Tobramycin
• Macrolides: Reversible, impair ion transport in SV
  • Clarithromycin, Erythromycin (high IV doses)
• Anti-malarials:
  • Quinine: Temporary tinnitus, vertigo
• Vancomycin: Rare, synergistic with gentamicin
	Chemotherapy agents
	• Platinoids:
	  • Cisplatin (OHCs, SV, spiral ganglion cells, and the vestibular system) 50% hearing toxicity, low vestibulotoxicity, toxic dose >200 mg/m^2
	  • Carboplatin: 15% hearing toxicity
	• Taxanes:
	  • Docetaxel, paclitaxel

Diuretics: Reversible • Furosemide (tinnitus) • Bumetanide	**NSAIDs and salicylates: Reversible** • Aspirin (temporary high-pitched tinnitus) • Indomethacin • Diclofenac
Others • Phenytoin	

3. Examination:
   - Otoscopy: Usually normal, but to rule out potential cholesteatoma or effusion
   - Tuning fork tests to confirm SNHL
   - Cranial nerve assessment: Demyelinating disease or brainstem pathology
   - Vestibular toxicity: Head thrust, dynamic visual acuity, caloric testing, rotation chair (sensitive early test)
4. Investigations:
   - Early detection/monitoring of those at risk
     - ASHA recommendations for baseline assessment <24 hrs after administration
     - Further tests based on patient symptoms or if child, an automatic follow-up

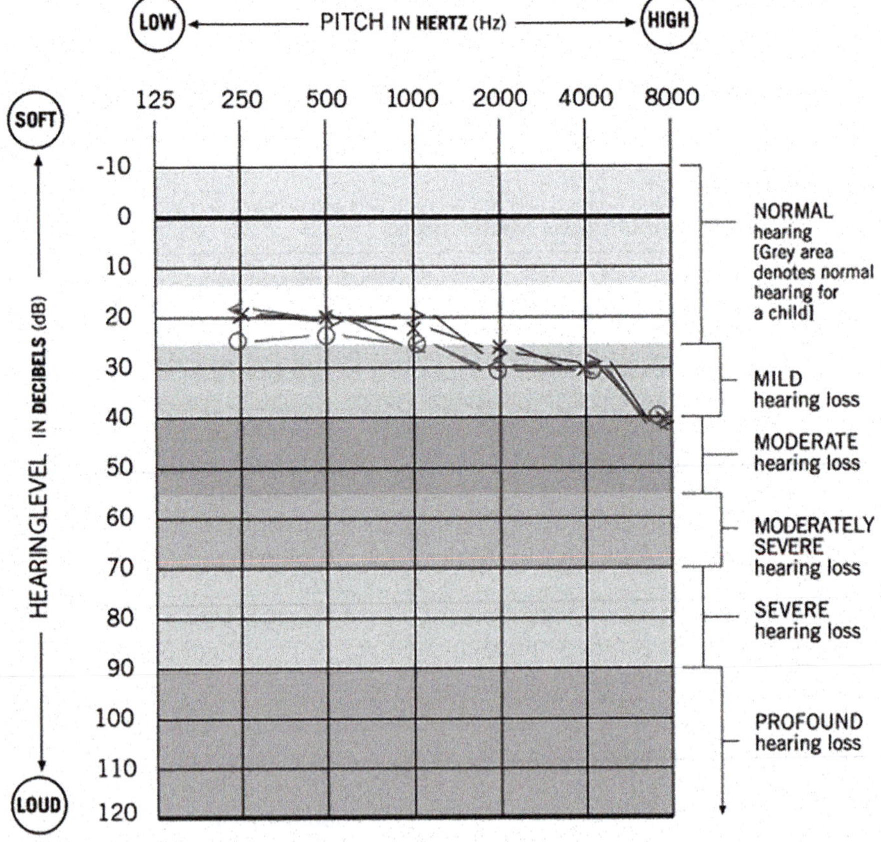

Figure 3.1 Pure tone audiogram demonstrating bilateral mild high frequency sensorineural hearing loss in keeping with presbyacusis.

- Baseline audiological investigations:
  - Objective: OAE, ABR, high-frequency audiometry
  - Subjective: VRA, PTA (depends on age)
- MRI if sensorineural asymmetry or alternate pathology

5. Management:
   - Conservative:
     - Omit offending agent: May improve hearing or halt progression
     - Tinnitus retraining therapy
     - Hearing aid trial in initial instance
     - Vestibular rehabilitation
   - Medical:
     - Sodium thiosulphate – protective medication: Reduced cisplatin-induced hearing loss Brock NEJM 2018
   - Cochlear implantation for profound pre-lingual deafness

Audiology

1. Key terms:
   - Frequency: Cycles/second = pitch
   - Intensity: Loudness
     - HL: HL based on reference of normal human hearing threshold for each frequency
     - SPL (sound pressure level): Based on absolute pressure measurement, hearing not linear so greater sound intensity in SPL needed for some frequencies to reach threshold; HL normalises these values
     - SL (sensation level): Relative to patient's threshold, important for speech testing
   - Interaural attenuation: Amount a signal is reduced when passing to the contra-lateral side
     - 60 dB for insert earphones
     - 40 dB for circumaural headphones (direct contact with skull, hence lower intensity required)
     - Must not exceed 0 dB for bone conduction, as assumption is that BC (test) = BC (non-test)
   - Speech testing:
     - Realistic representation of hearing due to presence of amalgamation of tones rather than one, complementary to PTA (only provides indication of absolute perceptual thresholds of tonal sounds)
     - Speech reception threshold (SRT): Measures lowest intensity level when patient can repeat 50% of common bisyllabic words e.g. baseball; this should correspond to PTA

    - Speech detection threshold: Lowest intensity level when patient can detect presence of speech, not necessarily bisyllabic words; used when SRT cannot be obtained
    - Word recognition/speech discrimination: Measures ability to repeat single syllabic words at suprathreshold level (approx. 40 dB above SRT)
    - Recruitment: Abnormal increase in loudness of sound, sign of sensory cochlear disorder
2. Masking: Isolation of non-test ear to prevent it from responding to signal
    - Noise is narrow band for pure tones or pink noise for speech
    - Crossover: Sound presented to the test ear is detected on the non-test side due to vibrations of the skull
    - Shadow curve: Thresholds for test ear reflect responses on non-test ear
    - Rule 1: AC mask if ≥40 dB difference between the AC (or 55 dB for inserts)
    - Rule 2: BC mask if ≥10 dB difference between AC in better ear and unmasked BC
    - Rule 3: AC mask if ≥40 dB difference between AC in better ear and unmasked BC
3. Acoustic reflex:
    - Stapedius muscle in middle ear contracts in response to an intense sound
        - Crossed vs uncrossed
        - CN VIII > cochlear nucleus > SOC (bilateral) > FN nucleus (bilateral) > stapedius
    - Pattern of abnormality helps identify site of lesion
    - Normal stapedial reflex threshold is 70–100 dB above the pure tone threshold
    - If suspect retrocochlear pathology, test acoustic reflex decay: Decreased auditory perception with sustained stimulus

Stapedial reflexes

Stapedial reflex absent in:

- Otosclerosis
- Any conductive loss
- Auditory neuropathy (OAE present: IHC/nerve dysfunction)
- Retrocochlear: Rollover phenomenon
- Facial nerve dysfunction

Present in:

- SSCD (helps with diagnosis to know that it is present)

4. Tympanometry: Measures function of TM, middle ear and acoustic reflex pathway
   - Immittance: General term that includes either admittance or impedance
   - Admittance: Ease of flow through system (most equipment measures admittance i.e. transmitted sound)
   - Acoustic impedance: Resistance to energy transfer (other equipment measures reflected sound)
     - Sum of friction, mass (contributes very little) and stiffness (main variable)
   - Compliance (mobility) = 1/impedance
     - Low-resistance (impedance) system will have free mobility (compliance) i.e. disarticulated ossicles
     - High-resistance system will result in poor mobility (low compliance) i.e. OME or otosclerosis
   - Tympanometry compliance changes against pressure within the EAC
     - Peak admittance when pEAC = pME
   - Ear canal volume: <1 mL in children and <2 mL in adults
   - Compliance: ~1.5 mL in adults, 0.5 mL in children (cm)
5. Electrocochleography: Measures electrical activity from cochlea and CN VIII
   - Gold standard for outer hair cell function
   - Utilised in endolymphatic hydrops
   - Recording of electrical potentials generated within cochlea and auditory nerve in response to wideband click stimuli
   - Probe on promontry (transtympanic), against tympanic membrane or in canal, click or tone burst stimuli introduced and electrical potentials recorded
   - Variables measured:
     - Cochlear microphonic (CM): AC microphonic potential, seen as cochlea is stimulated
     - Summation potential (SP): DC potential, current generated in hair cells
     - Compound action potential (CAP): Averaged activity of action potentials of CN VIII

       SP/CAP >0.45 is suggestive of Meniere's disease, syphilis, auditory nerve neurophonic
6. ABR/BAER:
   - Onset response and requires synchronous neural discharges to produce clear waveforms (seven waves)
   - Indications:
     - Threshold testing in difficult patients/malingering
     - Vestibular schwannoma diagnosis

    - Diagnosis of brainstem lesions
    - Intra-op monitoring
    - Newborn hearing screen – failed OAE
- Electrodes placed on forehead, vertex, mastoid or earlobe
- Seven waves measured NB only waves I, III and V present at birth
- Clicks or tone bursts introduced in ear (50/s) and electrodes measure ABR waves
    - Click rate varies between centres, in UK usually 45.1–49.1/sec (lower for tone bursts)

Retro-cochlear lesion audiometric findings:

Rollover phenomenon:	Reduction in speech/word recognition score with increasing intensity
Phonemic regression:	Disproportionate speech recognition when compared to pure tone thresholds
Acoustic reflex decay:	Decreased auditory perception with sustained stimulus

Symbols typically used in audiometry:

	Right	*Left*
Air unmasked	O	X
Air masked	Δ	□
Bone unmasked	<	>
Bone masked	[	]
Sound field	S	S
Aided	A	A

E. coli mnemonic:

Eight nerve:	Wave I
Cochlear nucleus:	Wave II
Olive (superior):	Wave III
Lateral lemniscus:	Wave IV
Inferior colliculus:	Wave V (largest wave)
Medial geniculate:	Wave VI
Auditory radiation:	Wave VII (Brodmann's area)

Hearing tests:

Type	*Description*	*Typical Age*
Neonatal hearing screening: Automated otoacoustic emissions, automated auditory brainstem response	AOAE: Sounds sent through earpiece placed in ear canal and microphone records the otoacoustic responses in response to sounds AABR: Electrodes attached to head (forehead, mastoid, shoulder), clicks via headphones	Contra-indications to screening: Atresia/ microtia, bacterial meningitis, cCMV, programmable shunt Well baby: Ideally within 4–5 weeks of birth; AOAE ± AABR NICU: AOAE and AABR If fail AABR → audiology referral within 4 weeks or by 44 weeks old
Visual reinforcement audiometry	Sounds presented to child which link to a visual award e.g. toy or computer screen lighting up	6 months–2.5 yrs
Play audiometry	Sounds via headphones or speakers; perform simple task when hear a sound e.g. put ball in bucket	1.5–5 yrs
Pure tone audiometry	Sounds via headphones; press button when hear sound	>5 yrs

Air Conduction Hearing Devices

1. Key concepts:
   - Benefit noticed when >30 dB loss over three frequencies (three subthreshold levels required for programming)
   - Acoustic gain: Amount of amplification provided by hearing aid, difference between input and output SPL (50 dB tone presented vs output of 80 dB = 30 dB gain)

    - High frequency average "HFA" gain: Average gain at 1000, 1600 and 2500 Hz
  - Harmonic distortion: Addition of frequencies not present in original sound
  - Saturation sound pressure: Max sound pressure the aid can produce
  - Dynamic range: Amount of amplification before sound becomes uncomfortable
  - Occlusion effect:
    - Perception of loudness of own voice as bone conducted sound is trapped by occlusive object
    - More common if normal hearing at low frequencies and poor hearing at high frequencies (occlusion effect at <500 Hz)
    - Managed by ear mould modifications (used less now due to advances in technology but still useful particularly in children)
      - ■ Non-occluding or open ear mould reduces low-frequency energy
      - ■ Treated by increasing venting: Hole in mould from EAC to the outside to reduce pressure sensation e.g. Libby Horn, "reverse horn"
  - ACHAs are readily available and inexpensive
    - Occlusive mould (50 dB or worse) i.e. moderate to severe HL
      - ■ Limit feedback
      - ■ Reduce loss of amplified sound
      - ■ Reduced ventilation, hence predispose to infections, modify with widened vents, hypoallergenic or softer moulds
    - Dome (open fit for 30–50 dB) i.e. mild-to-moderate HL
2. Types:
  - Behind the ear (BTE): Commonly used in NHS
  - Body sits behind ear, connected to ear mould via hollow tube
  - Induction coil for use with TV/telephones
  - Induction loop to remove background signals

  In the ear/in the canal (ITE, ITC, CIC): Degree of visibility of hearing aid (completely, barely visible, invisible)
  - Acrylic moulds conformed to patient's ear
  - High feedback rate due to proximity of microphone and transmitter
  - Ear canal acts as resonance chamber for sounds at 2 kHz, thus ITE aids are dampened at this frequency

  Extended wear hearing aid:
  - Air conduction device
  - For mild-to-moderate hearing loss
  - Increased gain, reduced feedback, reduced occlusion effect

  Contralateral routing of signal (CROS)/BiCROS:
  - Receiver (microphone) positioned on poorer hearing side
  - Transmitter placed on better ear
  - BiCROS: **Bilateral** hearing loss i.e. the better hearing ear is also impaired so amplification on better hearing side

Body worn aid (rarely used):

- For patients with dexterity issues (elderly)
- Powerful by way of size
- Large distance between receiver and transmitter so feedback is rarely problematic
- Clothing friction may cause interference

Bone conduction aids:

- Similar to body worn aids
- Output is via a bone conductor
- Not effective as not direct bone conduction (transcutaneous)

3. Implantable middle ear hearing aids (MEIs):
   - For moderate to severe CHL, SNHL or MHL where BCHDs and ACHAs are not suitable
   - Advantages: No occlusive effect, cosmetically discreet
   - Surgically implanted (fully or semi) within the middle ear e.g. vibrant usually on short process incus
   - Various approaches depending on type of MEI: Post-aural incision, bone bed, ± posterior tympanotomy
   - Partial implantation (MED-EL SOUNDBRIDGE) or total (Cochlear Carina)
     - MRI incompatible, although recent SOUNDBRIDGE models are 1.5T MRI conditional (not older versions e.g. VORP 502) – warn auditory sensations, discomfort, remove external components, do not use local transmitter coils
   - Expensive
   - Not suitable for retro-cochlear pathology or recurrent AOM
   - Can be charged or programmed transcutaneously

Components of hearing devices:

Microphone:	Acoustic energy converted to electrical energy
Amplifier/processor:	Electrical signal amplified and converted to acoustic energy
Transmitter:	Earphone or bone conductor
Power source:	On/off

Bone Conduction Hearing Devices

1. Key concepts:
   - Direct stimulation of the cochlea by transmitted vibrations via bones of the skull

- Components (see Figure 3.2)
    - Microphone: Converts sound to digital signal
    - Amplifier: Amplifies signal
    - Output receiver: Earphone or bone conductor. Signal converted back to analogue form
- Types:
    - Over skin drives or direct bone drives: Direct bone drives generally better outcome as skin can dampen sound pressure at higher frequencies
    - Direct bone drive divided into:
        - ■ Percutaneous device: Titanium screw osseointegrates into bone, abutment attaches external sound processor to screw (Cochlear Baha®)
            - o Osseointegration: New bone is deposited onto implanted material i.e. titanium
            - o Titanium has high tensile strength, corrosive resistance, biocompatible
            - o Transmission is passive, as the external aid is the only active component
            - o Infection, wound dehiscence, fixture loss, high complication rate for paediatric patients
        - ■ Passive transcutaneous device: Implanted beneath skin. External component attached by magnet (Cochlear® Baha Attract)
            - o Significant contact force required may cause pressure marks or skin pain – reduced device adherence
            - o Generate less gain than percutaneous devices
        - ■ Active transcutaneous device: Semi-implantable so vibratory energy does not need to be transmitted through skin (BONEBRIDGE Med-el® or Osia Cochlear®)
            - o Good functional outcomes through direct vibration of temporal bone
            - o Avoids complications of percutaneous abutment and gain loss of passive transcutaneous devices
- Fixture and abutment are MRI compatible

2. Indications for unilateral implantation: (NHSCB/D09/P/a 2013)
    - One of the following:
        - Permanent bilateral mixed or CHL
        - Unilateral CHL with ear canal stenosis unlikely to benefit from meatoplasty
        - Profound single-sided deafness
    - AND unsuitable for other treatments:
        - Congenital malformations of the outer/middle ear
        - Chronically discharging ear
        - Bilateral ossicular disease unable to be aided with ACHA or unsuitable for surgery

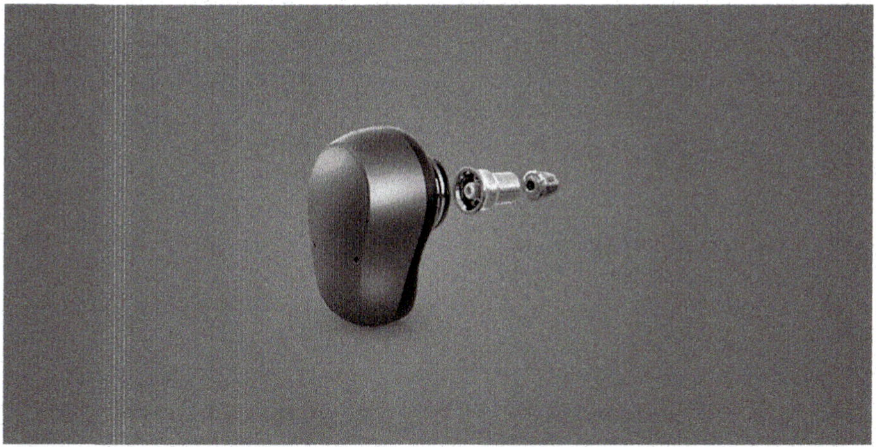

Figure 3.2 Photograph of bone conducting hearing system showing sound processor, abutment and fixture for osseointegration.

(Photograph courtesy of Oticon Medical.)

- AND audiological criteria:
  - BC threshold no worse than 45 dB HL (0.5, 1, 2, 3 kHz)
  - AC threshold no better than 40 dB HL
  - Speech discrimination score (SDS) >60% using a phonetically balanced word list
- AND:
  - Preoperative counselling, realistic expectations, prepared to maintain device
  - Keep area clean (on own or with assistance)
  - No contraindications

3. Contraindications:
   - Bone disease where skull is too thin to support BAHA implant e.g. osteogenesis imperfecta
   - <3 yrs. Usually 4–5 yrs to allow optimal bone thickness of 4 mm
     - Two-stage procedure with sleeper screw with 3-month interval to reduce OI failure
     - Microtia: Consider post-aural flaps, MDT for positioning, delay after 6 yrs (95% adult size)
   - Chronic skin disorders
   - Relative contraindications:
     - Psychiatric disease or psychological immaturity
     - Alcohol/drug abuse
4. Procedure:
   - Positioning: 5–6 cm from sup. aspect of EAC along temporal line (thicker bone, less muscle, no air cells)

  - Measure skin depth before LA (Lignospan [1:80,000 Adrenaline and 2% lidocaine])
  - Linear incision (or small flap in adults with soft tissue reduction) and cruciate incision on periosteum
  - 3 mm drill with spacer (1500 rpm) to assess depth; if so then proceed to 4 mm drill with spacer off
  - Then 4 mm countersink drill to widen
  - Insert 4 mm implant with abutment; Abutment depends on skin thickness (6, 9, 12 mm)
  - Post-op: Vicryl, dressing + healing cap; Dressing review 1/52; Installation at up to 3/12
5. Complications:
  - General (GA, pain, infection, bleeding, scarring, numbness to skin)
  - Failure of osseointegration, hence two sites implanted in children. Up to 15%
  - CSF leak: Rare
  - Bleeding: Sigmoid sinus trauma

Holgers grading

I: Erythema
II: Erythema, moistness
III: Granulation tissue
IV: Skin complications with implant removal

Cochlear Implantation

1. Background:
  - Structure See Figure 3.3
    - External device:
      - Microphone (above ear)
      - Processor (behind ear)
      - Transmitter (over internal component via magnet)
    - Implanted device:
      - Receiver/stimulator and electrode array
      - Multi-channel (12–22 electrodes depending upon manufacturer)
  - Improves speech recognition
  - Direct stimulation of cochlear nerve fibres in spiral ganglion
  - Criteria for implantation (TA566, 2019):
    - Minimum 3-month trial of ACHA

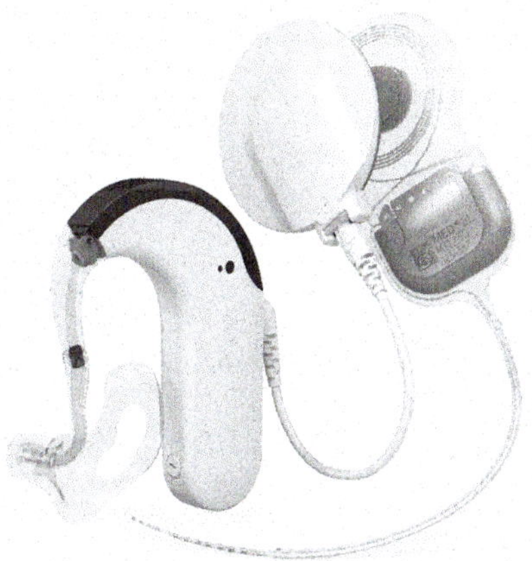

Figure 3.3 Photograph of hybrid electroacoustic stimulation device. Note the acoustic component (appears like a conventional air conduction device) plus the electrode array as per a typical cochlear implant device.

(Photograph courtesy of Med-El.)

- Thresholds: At or worse than 80 dB at ≥2 frequencies (500 Hz, 1,2,3,4 kHz) See Figure 3.4
- Children: Speech, language and listening skills not appropriate for age
- Adults: Phoneme score <50% on the Arthur-Boothroyd word test at 70 dBA

– Criteria for bilateral implantation:
  - Children:
    - ■ Pre-lingual deafness within 2 yrs
    - ■ Post-lingual deafness up to 10 yrs after onset of deafness (also adults)
    - ■ Meningitis, prior to cochlear ossification
  - Adults:
    - ■ Increased dependence on auditory stimuli (blindness, limited mobility) for spatial awareness

– Which side: If bilateral SNHL, side with most recent deafness or with poorest phenome score

2. History:
   – Age, and onset of deafness
   – Otological symptoms: Discharge, tinnitus, vertigo
   – Psychosocial impacts

   - PMH: Previous surgery, meningitis, ITU episodes (ototoxic medications), NICU/SCBU
   - DH: Ototoxic medications
3. Examination:
   - Otoscopy
   - Congenital malformations
4. Investigations:
   - Audiometric evaluation
   - CT/MRI for anatomy (middle ear/cochlea anomalies and presence of CN VIII)

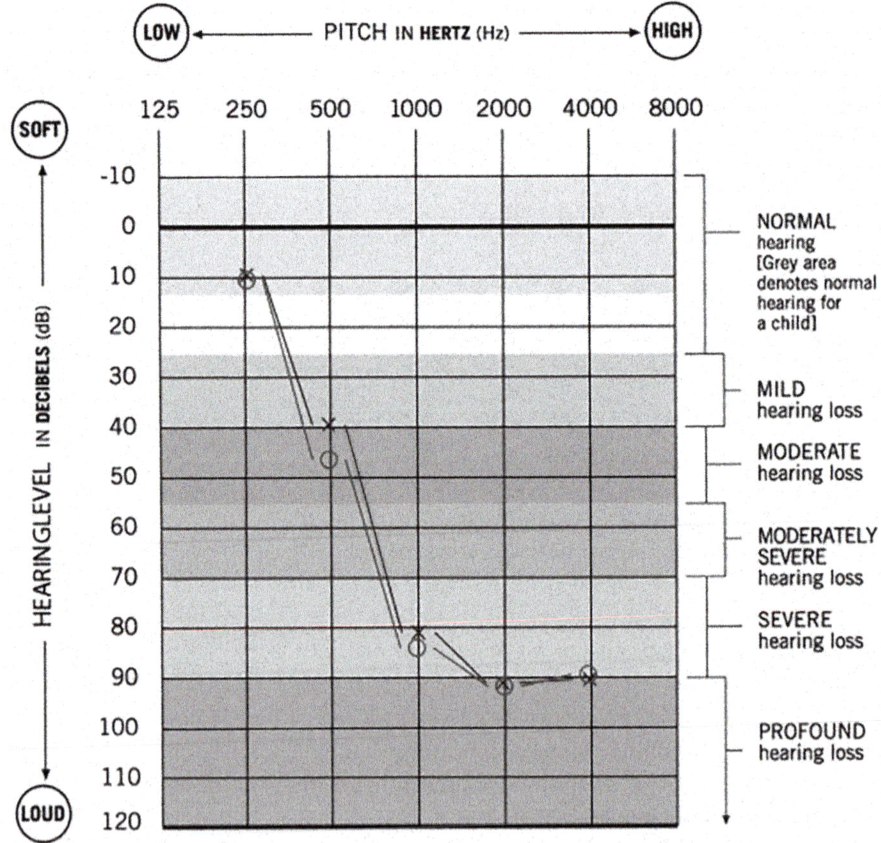

Figure 3.4 Pure tone audiogram showing profound mid and high frequency hearing loss with some preservation at low frequencies and potentially suitable for electroacoustic stimulation.

5. Management:
   - MDT approach: ENT, audiologists, paediatricians, geneticists
   - Procedure:
     - Post-aural incision (2 cm from sulcus) ± superior extension
     - Anterior, posterior, superior or inferiorly based periosteal flap
     - Cortical mastoidectomy + bone bed
     - Posterior tympanotomy
     - Cochleostomy or round window membrane (most common)
   - Contraindications:
     - Active CSOM
     - Agenesis of cochlea
     - Cochlear ossification (meningitis) – although consider insertion into second turn or SV
     - Retro-cochlear disease/NF2 (brainstem implant)
     - Absent CN VIII
   - Risks (as per mastoidectomy):
     - General (GA, pain, infection, bleeding, wound breakdown, implant extrusion)
     - Facial nerve paralysis
     - Taste disturbances
     - Dead ear
     - Tinnitus
     - Vertigo
     - CSF leak/meningitis
     - Perilymph gusher (increased with malformations)
     - Rare: Meningo/encephalocele
   - Cochlear implantation and middle ear effusions:
     - No intervention if serous fluid
     - Tympanostomy tubes for recurrent infections
     - AOM within 2 months should be treated aggressively
       - ■ Oral antibiotics for uncomplicated AOM outside 2/12 window with no inner ear malformation
       - ■ Parental antibiotics for those who do not meet criteria

Ossiculoplasty

1. Background:
   - Considered at time of primary surgery vs second stage procedure (significant or residual cholesteatoma, mucosal disease or ossicular disease i.e. fixation)
   - PORP vs TORP is dependent on presence of intact stapes suprastructure

- TORP is not used in the absence of a footplate (consider cartilage)
- Maximum ABG is 50–60 dB

Zollner-Wullstein classification:

Type 1: Myringoplasty (technically also requires examination of the ossicular chain)
Type 2: TM to incus/malleus remnant or restoration of lever mechanism (ISJ erosion)
Type 3: TM to stapes suprastructure
Type 4: TM to stapes footplate
Type 5: TM to LSCC (5a) or stapedotomy (5b)

- Successful ossiculoplasty is defined as post-op ABG ≤ 20 dB
- Belfast rule of thumb: Benefit achieved from OCR if post-operative thresholds are:
  - <30 dB or within 15 dB of contra-lateral ear
- Glasgow benefit plot:
  - Plot of pre-and post-operative mean air conduction thresholds
  - Provides visual representation of improvement post operatively
  - Normal hearing thresholds assumed to be 30 dB
    - Region 1: Normal bilateral hearing
    - Regions 2 and 3: 1 Normal hearing ear
    - Regions 4 and 6: Bilateral hearing loss but asymmetric
    - Region 5: Bilateral symmetrical hearing loss
  - Pre-op most patients fall in regions 2, 5 and 6 (not 3 as non-operated ear should not be worse unless it is a non-hearing preservation procedure)

2. History
   - Hearing loss duration, progression, onset
   - Questions related to causes (see box)
3. Examination
   - Otoscopy
4. Investigations
   - PTA
   - Speech tests
   - Tympanometry
     - As = fixation (dec compliance)
     - Ad = Hypermobility, e.g. discontinuity (inc compliance)
     - B = Effusion (normal canal volume)/perf (high canal volume)
     - C = normal pressure, shifted to left

5. Management:

Reconstructive Options	
Synthetic	*Autologous*
• PORP (partial ossicular replacement prosthesis) • TORP (total ossicular replacement prosthesis) • OtoMimix NB TORP and PORP are MRI safe (newer prostheses)	• Cartilage • Interposition (incus) grafts (prone to necrosis and fusion)

6. Evidence:
   - See Yu et al. PORP vs TORP meta-analysis. EAOS 2013; 270(12): 3005–3017
     - PORP hearing outcomes significantly better (and more predictable) than TORP
     - Lower extrusion rates
     - ABG to <20 dB in 70% PORP vs 50% TORP

Causes of hearing loss:

- Conductive hearing loss:
  - Outer ear:
    - Anotia/microtia
    - EAC atresia
    - Exostosis, osteoma
    - Wax
    - FB
    - Malignancy e.g. SCC
  - Middle ear:
    - TM perf
    - OME
    - Retraction
    - Otosclerosis
    - Ossicular fixation: Acquired vs congenital
    - Ossicular discontinuity: Trauma, inflammation, tumour
    - Cholesteatoma
    - Tympanosclerosis

Tympanometry

Tympanometry measures ME *immittance* = impedance + admittance

- Impedance: "resistance" to sound input
- Admittance: "ease" of sound input
- Immittance greatest when EAC: ME pressure same – maximal compliance
- Allows measure of ME pressure
- Allows measure of EAC effective volume (detect perforations)

Presbyacusis

1. Background:
   - ? Atrophy of stria vascularis (SV)? Loss of sensory hair cells? Loss of neural tissue? See Table 3.2
   - Age-related hearing loss (typically affects basal turn IHCs first)
   - Clinical diagnosis based on history with no other pathology to account for loss of hearing
   - Schuknecht classification not really supported by animal or latest data
     - K Steel: Presbyacusis presents with metabolic, neural, and/or sensory phenotypes
2. History: Used to rule out other pathology
   - Timing/onset i.e. age (usually older patients)

Table 3.2 Schuknecht Classification

Type	*Features*
Sensory	• Affects organ of Corti • Steep slope • Normal SD (loss above speech frequency, as basal cochlea affected first
Neural (nerve/spiral ganglion)	• 50% cochlear neuronal loss • Flatter audiogram • Disproportionate drop in SD for loss of hearing
Stria (stria vascularis)	• SV supplies entire cochlea, hence all frequencies affected, hence flat audiogram • SD preserved
Mechanical/cochlear conductive	• Thickening of basilar membrane • Down sloping or upward sloping towards HF • Normal SDS

   - Progression: Slow gradual decline in hearing
   - Lateralisation: Usually bilateral
   - Infective symptoms
   - Tinnitus/vertigo
   - Barotrauma
   - PMH: Systemic causes (DM, MS, SLE)
   - DH: Ototoxic medications
   - FH: Genetics
   - SH: Occupation (NIHL/acoustic trauma)
3. Examination:
   - Otoscopy usually normal
   - Neuro-otological examination if alternative diagnosis likely i.e. associated vertigo
4. Investigations:
   - Audiogram demonstrates the above patterns
   - Blood tests (rarely indicated): VDRL, HIV, Lyme's disease, ESR, ANA, ANCA, RF (autoimmune pathology), genetic testing (multifactorial genes, if audiovestibular loss then consider DFNA9)
5. Management:
   - Conservative:
     - Hearing rehabilitation as hearing loss is associated with low QOL, depression and social isolation
     - Hearing aids (ACHA) for minimum 6/12
   - Surgical:
     - BCHA
     - MEI
     - CI if criteria met
6. Differential diagnoses:
   - Autoimmune hearing loss: Immune mediated inner damage and deposition of immune complexes within inner ear:
     - Examples: RA, Cogan's, SLE, PAN
     - Usually present at younger age
     - Fluctuating (with disease)
     - Rapid compared to presbyacusis
     - Bilateral
     - Associated with tinnitus and vertigo as well as fullness
     - Treatment: Refer to Rheumatologist, Prednisolone (60 mg/day), with tapering if improvement – another feature of AIHL
     - Often need long-term immunosuppression
   - Noise-induced hearing loss
   - Ototoxicity
   - Genetic hearing loss e.g. DFNA9
   - Infective: Lyme, syphilis etc.

Speech tests:

Speech reception threshold (SRT):

- Level at which bisyllabic words heard 50% of time

Speech discrimination score (SDS):

- % of monosyllabic words heard at 20–40 dBSL above. Can also use sentence tests which also test top-down processing
- PBmax: Maximum monosyllabic word recognition score with increasing intensity, should be 100% with CHL

Sudden Sensorineural Hearing Loss

1. Background:
   - Rule of 3s: ≥30 dB HL at 3 frequencies, over 3 days
     - 1/3 partial recovery, 1/3 full recovery, 1/3 no recovery
   - Worse prognosis: Advanced age, late presentation/delay to treatment, profound or high- frequency HL, vertigo
   - Cause unknown in 85–95% of cases

Idiopathic (60%)		
Congenital:	Aminoglycoside sensitivity (mitochondrial)	
Traumatic:	Iatrogenic/surgery, temporal bone fracture, barotrauma e.g. scuba diving, acoustic trauma e.g. explosion, noise	
Medications:		
	Quinines	
	NSAIDs:	Aspirin, ibuprofen, naproxen
	Aminoglycosides:	Gentamicin or tobramicin
	Loop diuretics:	Furosemide
	Chemotherapeutics:	Cisplatin, carboplatin
	Antiseptics:	Chlorhexidine, ethyl alcohol
Infection:	AOM, Herpes, CSOM,	
Inflammatory:	TORCH	
Autoimmune:	Cogan, SLE, RA, Behcet	
Systemic:	DM, CVA, MS	
Neoplastic:	CPA lesion (meningioma, epidermoid, VS)	

2. History:
   - Timing: Abrupt drop or progressively over days
   - Unilateral/bilateral

   - Associated symptoms: Fullness, tinnitus, vertigo
   - History of trauma
   - PMH: Cardiovascular risk factors, autoimmune disease
   - DH: Ototoxic medications
3. Examination:
   - Otoscopy to rule out middle ear disease
   - Neurological examination (multiple CN involvement implies systemic cause i.e. MS)
4. Investigations:
   - Haemotological investigations only in event of high suspicion of i.e. autoimmune pathology
     - U&Es, LFTs, FBC, ESR, CRP, VDRL, ANA, RF, ANCA, Lyme's serology
   - Baseline audiogram
   - MRI IAM to rule out retro-cochlear pathology
   - CT or ABR if MRI contra-indicated
5. Management:
   - Conservative: Hearing rehabilitation
     - Hearing aids:
       - ACHA: BEA, BCHA, CROS/BiCROS (most cost effective)
   - Medical: Controversial treatments with low-level evidence
     - Carbogen as vasodilator 5% CO_2, 95% O_2 (limited data/evidence exists)
     - Hyperbaric oxygen (HBO)
     - Oral prednisolone 1 mg/kg max 60 mg for 7/7 within 2/52 (ideally 72 hrs)
       - Tapering only recommended if:
         - 40 mg daily for >1/52
         - Treatment overall >3/52
         - Repeated treatments, again amounting to 3/52
     - IT steroid, particularly if failed course of PO, diabetic or risk factors, within 2–6/52 of onset
       - Role as primary, combination or salvage treatment, but low-level evidence
     - Risks of steroids: Counsel prior to initiation and consider PPI prophylaxis (especially if NSAIDs)
       - Endocrine: Cushing's syndrome, elevated BMs/DM in long-term use
       - Immune: Suppression with increased risk of infections
       - Psych: Low mood/depression/acute psychosis
       - CVS: HTN
       - Gastro: PUD
       - MSK: Osteoporosis, avascular necrosis of hip
     - Cochlear implant for single-sided deafness

6. Evidence:
   - Cochrane (2013): Steroids for idiopathic SSNHL
     - Conflicting evidence due to lack of robust data with low numbers. Three trials, one showing benefit
     - Earlier intervention demonstrates favourable outcomes (intervention timing not discussed)
     - Limited efficacy after 3 weeks
   - See Gao et al. Meta-analysis: Combined IT and systemic use of steroids for ISSHL. Eur Arch Otolaryngol 2016; 273(11): 3699–3711
     - Evidence for dual modality therapy

Tinnitus

1. Background:
   - Perception of sound in absence of stimulus
   - 10% prevalence, increasing with age (may be higher than this, British Tinnitus Association quote 1 in 8 people)
   - 80% will have measurable hearing loss
   - 10% report intrusiveness
   - Divided into:

Subjective	*Objective*
• More common than objective • Associated with HFHL (3–5 Hz)	• Caused by internal body sound (usually vascular) • Exacerbated by a CHL • Sometimes pulse synchronous • Consider middle ear muscle myoclonus, palatal myoclonus

Causes:

Hearing loss: Ototoxicity, presbyacusis, NIHL

Vascular:

1. IIH
2. Venous outflow obstruction (e.g. styloid)
3. Venous other: High jugular bulb, dehiscent sigmoid, emissary vein
4. AVM: Pulse synchronous
5. Vascular bruits/hums: Atherosclerosis or nearby vessels such as high riding jugular bulb or persistent stapedial artery

6. Vascular tumour:	Glomus tympanicum
7. Systemic:	Hypertension, hyperthyroidism, blood flow changes during pregnancy
Mechanical:	
1. Patulous ET:	Autophony, hyponasality. Causes include radiation, weight loss, CVA. Consider hydration, injection with bulking agents, grommets, cartilage graft, oestrogen drops
2. Palatal myoclonus:	Consider muscle relaxants, botox
3. Tensor tympani/stapedius:	Low-frequency tinnitus, accentuated by external sound. Tinnitus may be synchronous with TM movement or with audible clicking in ear canal

2. History:
   - Unilateral vs bilateral
   - Timing: Intermittent vs constant, daytime vs nocte
   - Character of tinnitus: Pulsatile, ringing, buzzing
   - Exacerbation (stress) and alleviation (head positioning)
   - Associated hearing loss, discharge, vertigo
   - PMH: CV risk factors
   - DH: Salicylates, ototoxic medications (see SSNH)
   - SH: Intrusiveness: Effects on social life, sleeping, low mood, occupation (NIHL)
3. Examination:
   - Otoscopy to elicit middle ear cause for tinnitus
     - Check for patulous ET
   - Auscultation of neck for bruits
   - Oral cavity for palatal myoclonus
   - Check for pulse synchronicity
4. Investigations:
   - Audiogram + tympanometry
   - MRI if unilateral symptoms, localising signs, pulsatile tinnitus (or MRA) or audiometric SNHL indication (NICE guidelines NG98):
     - ≥15 dB asymmetry at 2 neighbouring frequencies using test frequencies 0.5, 1, 2, 4, 8 kHz
5. Management:
   - Conservative:
     - Medication eradication: NSAIDs, aspirin, aminoglycosides, anti-hypertensive

    - Caffeine, smoking cessation
    - CBT (best evidence base)/TRT
    - Relaxation
    - Hearing aids
    - Masking: White noise centred (notched or peaked) around tinnitus frequency
  - Medical management (none of these likely to be initiated by ENT):
    - Benzodiazepines
    - Tricyclic anti-depressants
    - Carbamazepine
  - Surgical:
    - BCHA for single-sided deafness
    - Cochlear implantation not funded for unilateral hearing loss in UK currently
    - Resurfacing of sigmoid sinus
    - Interventional radiology stenting/coiling for venous obstruction, or styloid surgery
    - Specialist surgical intervention for pulsatile tinnitus

Noise-Induced Hearing Loss

1. Background:
   - Hearing loss due to acoustic trauma/over-exposure:
     - Can be temporary: Temporary threshold shift (TTS), typically improves within 2–3 days but may take 2 weeks
     - Repeated TTSs may lead to a permanent threshold shift (PTS)
     - Even PTS may lead to synaptopathy, which can affect speech comprehension (Charles Lieberman's work)
   - 3, 4, 6 kHz dip characteristic See Figure 3.5
   - Due to position of cochlea, basal turn affected before apical turn (higher frequencies affected more than lower)
   - Resonance frequency of middle ear and ossicles: 1–4 kHz, hence maximal energy transfer and notching
   - Acoustic reflex is triggered by noise >90 dB
     - Latency of acoustic reflex = 10 ms
     - Hence, sudden insult will reach cochlea prior to reflex activation
     - Result is immediate; irreversible damage
   - >140 dB single insult: Ossicular or inner ear damage (hair cell damage from ruptured membranes and mixing of peri and endolymph)
   - >180 dB: TM rupture and fracture of ossicles
   - The control of noise at work regulations 2005 sets standard for employers
2. History:
   - Always focus on broad history as may be multifactorial

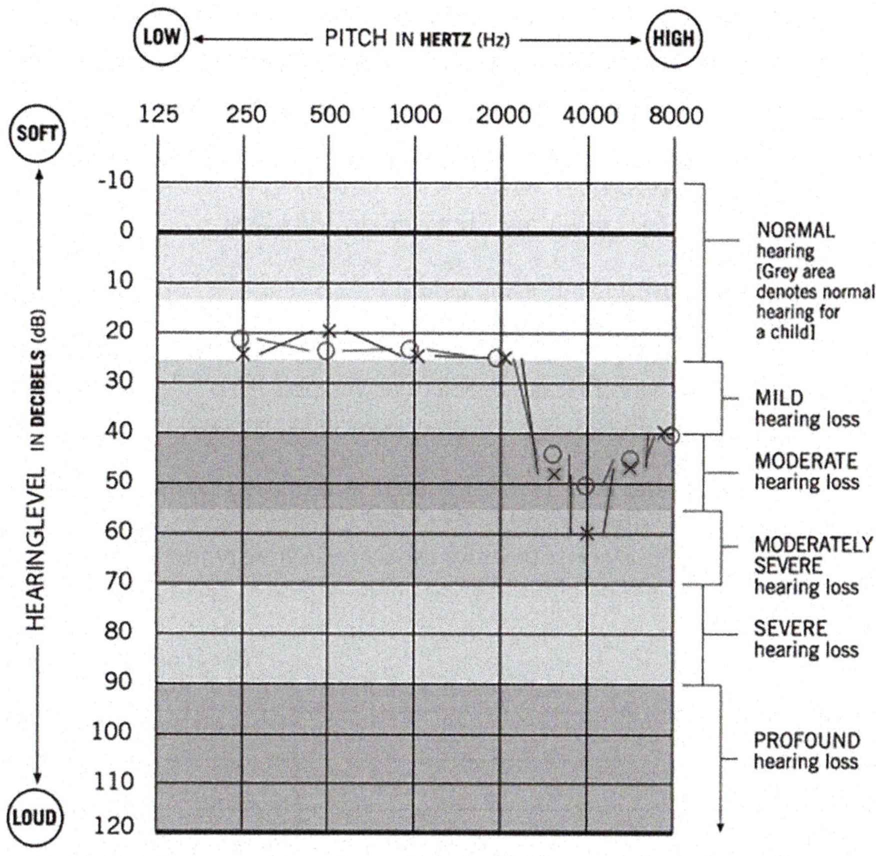

Figure 3.5 Pure tone audiogram showing notches at 4kHz, worse in the left ear than the right, typical of noise induced hearing loss. Depending on the previous noise exposure the notch may be more prominent at another frequency or difficult to distinguish within the context of previous noise exposure, aging or other causes of hearing damage.

- PC:
  - Onset: Sudden, gradual
  - Associated tinnitus or vertigo
  - Infective symptoms
- PMH:
  - Previous meningitis/ITU admissions
  - Previous otological history (e.g. ototoxicity, radiotherapy to H&N)
- DH: Potential ototoxic medications
- FH: Of hearing loss? Congenital? Otosclerosis? predisposition to NIHL (several candidate genes)
- SH: Occupation/repeated loud noise exposure, shooting/nightclubs

3. Examination:
   – Otoscopy to assess for perforation (usually unremarkable)
   – Cranial nerve assessment
4. Investigations:
   – Audiometry/tympanometry
   – Acoustic reflexes
   – If asymmetric hearing loss, then consider MRI IAM
5. Management:
   – Conservative: Usually main option
     - Prevention of further hearing loss
     - Occupational intervention: Control of Noise at Work Regulations 2005 (part of Health & Safety at Work Act 1974)
       - Measured in dB and given A weighing (average) or C weighting (peak)
       - Lower limit is the threshold to risk assess (if over 85 dBA or 137 dBC)
       - Upper limit is the threshold where hearing protection is required
       - Exposure limit is the maximum employees' exposure

	Average Exposure (dBA)	*Peak Sound Pressure (dBC)*
Lower limit	80	135
Upper limit	85	137
Exposure limit	87	140

     - Can consider hearing aid devices if significant disability
     - Tinnitus retraining therapy
   – May benefit from steroids: Acoustic trauma: Low-level evidence
     - Offered up to 3 weeks post-insult, but the earlier the better
     - Controversy between Methylprednisolone and Dexamethasone for ITSI
     - Intra-tympanic presumed better as salvage modality
     - Dual modality potentially better than single modality (repeated IT injections up to maximum of three)

TTS and PTS:

NIHL is damage to hearing as a result of **acoustic overexposure** OHC initially but potential cascade of damage.

TTS = temporary threshold shift

PTS = permanent threshold shift
(increased intensity, longer duration)
TTS is worsening of hearing after acoustic exposure that resolves over period of days.

Non-Organic Hearing Loss

1. Background:
   - Non-organic hearing loss: Apparent loss with no physical problem to explain
     - Includes malingering (intentional) and conversion disorders (unintentional)
   - Suspicion raised based on audiological findings:
     - Irregularities between tests (test retest, between PTA and speech, OAEs and reflexes)
     - Unmasked BC can never be worse than best ear AC
     - Unmasked AC between 2 ears of >40 dB suspicious as unlikely due to interaural cross over
     - Half word answers on balanced spondees
   - A high index of suspicion must be held, particularly if claiming compensation
2. History:
   - Detailed account of hearing loss
   - Exclude organic problems: SOL, infections, trauma, surgery, autoimmune
   - Fluctuating degree
   - FOCUS ON SOCIAL Hx
     - Depression, anxiety
     - Life stresses e.g. school/work
     - Medication or treatments
3. Examination:
   - Physical examination usually normal
   - Conversational hearing performance better than would be suggested by PTA
4. Investigations:
   - Initial assessment may provide some information:
     - There may be an apparent difference in hearing in clinic against PTA findings
   - Tests include:
     - Subjective:
       - PTA and tympanometry:
         - Inconsistent results, typically with a flat audiogram, with thresholds 40–50 dB

    - o Patient may deny hearing stimulus when bone conduction is unmasked (should hear in contra-lateral cochlea which has normal hearing thresholds)
  - ■ Speech audiometry:
    - o Patients will find it difficult to exaggerate impairment compared to PTA
  - ■ Stenger test:(unilateral hearing loss)
    - o Usually tuning fork or more often audiometry
    - o Two tuning forks placed an equal distance apart and tuning fork distance reduced in "affected" ear
    - o If true hearing loss, then the normal ear will not be masked and patient should still hear stimulus in normal ear
    - o In NOHL, they will deny hearing in better ear, as the tuning fork on the contra-lateral ear masks the better ear
  - ■ Lombard's test (L = Loud):
    - o Principle is that in a busy environment, an individual will raise their voice
    - o Headphones placed within the EAC and patient is asked to read a text
    - o With a true hearing loss, the patient will not change the intensity of their voice as background noise intensity is increased, whereas in a NOHL, they will
  - ■ Erhardt's test (E = Ear):
    - o Occluding the EAC of the normal ear will dampen sound by 30 dB, but patient should still hear voice of the tester
    - o In NOHL, patient will deny they can hear anything with the normal ear occluded
  - ■ Chimani-Moos:
    - o Modified Weber test, and works on canal-occlusion theory
    - o Patient should hear better with tuning fork on vertex with good ear occluded but will deny this in NOHL
  - ■ Delayed speech feedback:
    - o Patient reads aloud, and this is then played back into the affected ear (delayed)
    - o In NOHL, patient will stutter or hesitate, whereas in true organic hearing loss, they will continue to read
- Objective:
  - ■ Acoustic reflexes: See "Audiology" section
    - o The stapedial reflex threshold is usually 70 dB above pure tone threshold
    - o NOHL is unlikely, but this can be variable with recruitment (disproportionate loudness with increased intensity)

- Otoacoustic emissions:
  - o Are normal in auditory neuropathy and absent in middle ear disease such as glue ear
  - o Can distinguish between cochlear and retro-cochlear pathology
  - o Microphone in EAC measures sound generated by outer hair cells in response to auditory stimuli
  - o Generated by Organ of Corti under normal conditions (30 dBSPL)
  - o Click stimuli (wide band) or pure tones (narrow band)
    - – Spontaneous and stimulus frequency OAE are of no clinical use
    - – Evoked (occur after stimuli):
      - Transient evoked OAE: 20 ms after click stimuli (84 dBSPL) or tone
      - Response at multiple frequencies 700 Hz to 4 kHz
      - Present if HT 20 dB or better
      - Neonatal screening use
    - – Distortion product (DPOAE): 2 simultaneous pure tones (55, 65 dBSPL) at 2 frequencies
      - Using more than 1 frequency stimulates more aspects of basilar membrane
      - Unreliable for determining thresholds
      - For HFHL (1–8 kHz), hence used for NIHL and ototoxicity
- ABR:
  - o Requires masking along with cortical evoked response audiometry
  - o If HT <60 dB, may not get traced
  - o Recording activity of cochlear nerve and CNS response to auditory stimulus
  - o Electrodes placed on forehead, vertex, mastoid or earlobe
  - o *E. coli* mnemonic: See "Audiology" section
  - o Cortical or MLR electrophysiological responses

5. Management
   - – Explanation and reassurance. May not be well received by patient

Chronic Otitis Media

1. Background:
   - – Long-term inflammatory disorder of the middle ear
   - – Two distinct types:
     - Mucosal: Due to TM perforation and subsequent inflammation of ME mucosa. Sub-classify as active mucosal COM (aka CSOM) or inactive (perforation)

    - Squamous: Due to retraction of TM, associated with formation of cholesteatoma. Sub-classify as active (cholesteatoma) or inactive (retraction)
  - Definition of CSOM: Chronic inflammation of the middle ear and mastoid cavity, which presents with recurrent otorrhoea through a tympanic perforation, for over 6 weeks
2. History:
  - Duration, onset, progression of symptoms
  - Headaches (if suspected acute complications)
  - Hearing loss
  - Otorrhoea
  - Tinnitus
  - Previous surgery, grommets, eustachian tube dysfunction
  - History of AOM, ear trauma, glue ear
  - Impact upon school/work and language development
3. Examination:
  - Otoscopy (bilateral)
    - Valsalva – TM elevates?
    - Contralateral ear health –? eustachian tube dysfunction
  - Post-nasal space
  - Post-auricular swelling
  - Facial paralysis, vertigo
  - Signs of intracranial infection
4. Investigations:
  - PTA
  - Tympanometry both ears
  - CT (not warranted for retractions only)
5. Management:
  - Conservative: Watch and wait or hearing aids
    - Self-cleaning
    - Hearing stable
    - Valsalva manoeuvre including Otovent balloon
    - Water precautions
  - Surgical
    - Grommet/T-tube to ventilate middle ear
    - Cartilage tympanoplasty ± ossiculoplasty
      - Bone cement or prosthesis for long process of incus to stapes head
      - PORP
      - TORP
    - Pit-falls of surgery
      - Does not address underlying eustachian tube dysfunction so consider combining with ET dilatation

- Tympanoplasty rates are lower in children if recurrent AOM or eustachian tube dysfunction (think craniofacial anomaly, Down's syndrome, Cleft palate)
- Success rate increases with age until 11 yrs old
- Wait for adenoid pad to start regressing (6 yrs) or regressed (10 yrs)

Indications for CT:

1. Mastoid pneumatisation
2. Sigmoid sinus position
3. Jugular bulb position
4. Tegmen position
5. CN VII dehiscence
6. Ossicles
7. SCC fistula
8. Disease extent

Tympanic Membrane Retractions

1. Background:
   - Three factors are thought to cause retraction
     - Negative middle ear pressure due to eustachian tube dysfunction
     - Tympanic membrane weakening:
       - Previous trauma/perforation/grommets
       - Pars flaccida has a less organised middle TM (fibrous) layer, which predisposes it to retraction
       - The postero-superior quadrant of the TM has a weaker middle layer
     - Increased surface area of tympanic membrane:
   - Seen in 25% of children, with unilateral > bilateral, and common in patients with cleft palate
   - Can result in bony erosion (scutum or ossicles) and keratin accumulation due to interrupted migration of epithelium
2. History:
   - Many are asymptomatic
   - Those that do present, are due to hearing loss, whether due to the retraction or due to ossicular erosion
   - There may be evidence of recurrent discharge if there is formation of cholesteatoma

3. Examination:

Grading as follows:

	Tos (pars flaccida)	Sade (pars tensa)
Grade 1:	Dimpling	Mild retraction
Grade 2:	Onto malleus neck	ISJ adhesion
Grade 3:	Scutum erosion	Promontory, non-adhesive
Grade 4:	Frank cholesteatoma	Promontory, adhesive

4. Management:
   - Conservative:
     - Aural hygiene and observation with regular suction of any keratin deposits
     - Autoinflation, although benefits are temporary
     - Use of hearing aid devices
   - Medical:
     - Nasal decongestants, although evidence is minimal. Topical aural therapy for recurrent infections
   - Surgical:
     - Grommet insertion ± LASER stiffening of TM
     - Balloon tuboplasty: Efficacy being assessed at present by Cochrane collaborative
     - Tympanoplasty: *Zollner-Wullstein classification*
       - ■ Resection of retraction pocket, assessment of ossicular chain, removal of cholesteatoma, reconstruction with temporalis fascia/biodesign ± cartilage reinforcement. The likelihood of success is reduced in bilateral retraction

Type 1:	Myringoplasty (with inspection of ossicular chain)
Type 2:	TM to incus/malleus remnant or *restoration of lever mechanism* (i.e. discontinuity between ISJ)
Type 3:	TM to stapes suprastructure
Type 4:	TM to stapes footplate
Type 5:	TM to LSCC (5a) or stapedotomy (5b): Creation of a third window

5. Investigations:
   - PTA/tympanometry may demonstrate a conductive hearing loss with a flat or shallow trace
   - If evidence of frank cholesteatoma, then CT scan of the temporal bones:

  - Advantages: Mainly anatomical knowledge and potential planning of surgery
    - Position of dura, sigmoid sinus, ossicular/scutum erosion, mastoid aeration, presence of LSSC fistula, demonstrate dehiscence of facial nerve
    - This will determine approach. If low dura and anterior sigmoid sinus, then a CAT is out of the question
    - If the mastoid is well aerated, then a limited atticotomy may be undertaken potentially
  - Disadvantages:
    - False reassurance and radiation exposure, particularly in children, with an increased lifetime risk of malignancy

6. Miscellaneous:
   - Belfast rule of thumb: Patient perceives benefit if thresholds increased to 30 dB or within 15 dB of contra-lateral ear
   - Glasgow benefit plot: Audit tool, with average thresholds plotted for non-operated ear (X axis) against operated ear (Y axis). A further plot is then made following surgery
7. Evidence:
   - See Nankivell et al. 2010: 2 RCTs, but no evidence to support or refute the role of surgery in retraction pockets

Tympanic Membrane Perforation

1. Background:
   - Tympanic membrane perforations are common in both adults and children
   - Approximately, 85% of traumatic perforations will heal on their own in 6–8 weeks (advise water precautions in the meantime, antibiotics not needed unless dirty/infected)
2. History:
   - Frequent discharge or infections
   - Pain
   - Vertigo
   - Other ear hearing or hearing aid user?
   - Previous surgery/trauma
   - PMH
   - Interests and hobbies/occupation
3. Examination:
   - Both ears
4. Investigation:
   - PTA/tymps
     - ET function in contralateral ear

5. Management:
   - Conservative → medically unfit, asymptomatic
     - Hearing aid
     - Education → water precaution
   - Medical
     - Aural toilet
     - Topical drops
   - Surgery
     - Myringoplasty
       - Endoscopic or microscopic
       - Technique dependant on size and site
         - Plug or patch technique for small ones e.g. fat/cartilage butterfly
         - TF/perichondrium/cartilage/Biodesign graft underlay
         - Push through technique (endoscopic or microscopic)
         - Lateral overlay
6. Evidence:
   - Meta-analysis: Jalali et al. Comparison of cartilage with temporalis fascia tympanoplasty: A meta-analysis of comparative studies. Laryngoscope 2017; 127(9): 2139–2148
     - Cartilage tympanoplasty favoured TF for integration rate
     - Hearing outcomes were the same
   - In children:
     - Depends on sx
     - Conventional wisdom has been that it is preferable to delay to age 10–12, but there is no statistical evidence to support this. However, it is potentially prudent to wait until the contralateral ear has normalised as this is associated with improved outcomes (Hardman et al. Tympanoplasty for chronic tympanic membrane perforation in children: systematic review and meta-analysis. Otology & Neurotology 2015; 36(5): 796–804)
       - Improved ET function
       - Have to balance this with ages children keen to swim

Cholesteatoma

1. Background:
   - Benign keratinising squamous cell cyst + keratin core (up to 15 epithelial layers) causing localised infection and bony erosion
   - CHL through destruction of ossicles
   - Complications:
     - LSSC fistula (most common complication)
     - CN paralysis (tympanic segment of CN VII)
     - Intracranial complications (1:200 lifetime risk), same as AOM (intra/extra-cranial)

	Congenital Cholesteatoma	*Acquired Cholesteatoma*
Location	Anterior-superior mesotympanum	Post epitympanum > Post mesotympanum
Theory	Epidermoid (nest cells in foetus)	Primary/secondary (see below)
Age	4.5 yrs	Any age

- Locations: Temporal bone, skull base and meninges and external auditory canal
- Congenital: White mass, with no history of surgery or discharge. Squamous epithelium trapped during embryogenesis
- Acquired theories:
  - Primary:
    - Eustachian tube dysfunction:
      - Retraction pocket theory. Mainly within pars flaccida, due to dysfunctional epithelial migration
  - Secondary:
    - Implantation: From surgery/trauma
    - Metaplasia: Chronic infection leads to metaplastic change in middle ear epithelium
    - Papillary: Migration through pars flaccida following infection
    - Migration: Through existing perforation, usually marginal

2. History:
   - Recurrent infections, duration and number
   - Hearing loss, tinnitus, balance problems, facial weakness
   - Progressive headaches – ?impending intracranial complication
   - Nasal symptoms
   - Impact on behaviour and educational performance
   - PMH: Previous surgery (grommets), ETD
3. Examination:
   - Otoscopy: Perforation and retraction (see retracted TM section for grades), discharge, typically arises in attic defect (N.B. Tos classification for pars flaccida defects)
   - CN examination: CN VII palsy
   - Vestibular exam: Fistula test, head thrust
4. Investigations:
   - PTA: Affected and better hearing ear – most likely CHL or mixed
     - SNHL if cochlea breached
   - CT TB to support diagnosis:
     - Anatomical evaluation:
       - Low tegmen, high jugular bulb, pneumatisation (suitability for CWU)
       - Dehiscent facial nerve, LSSC fistula

        - ■ Scutum erosion, long process of incus erosion (tenuous blood supply)
        - ■ Prussak's space: Area between pars flaccida and malleus neck
  - Recurrence can be assessed with MRI: Non-EPI DWMRI (>2 mm cholesteatoma)
5. Management:
   - Only curative treatment is surgery but in elderly/unfit may be managed conservatively
   - Front to back or back to front, CWU or CWD, endoscopic or microscopic or combination
   - OCR dependent on confidence of disease clearance
   - Mastoid obliteration may reduce recurrence. Unlikely improve sound properties unless perforation present
   - Discharging cavity: Recurrence, high facial ridge, inadequate saucerisation, large cavity, TM perforation
   - Mastoidectomy:
     - Facial nerve monitor: 1 mA max, limit to 0.25–0.5 mA on the nerve directly
     - McEwan's triangle: Antrum is 1.5 cm deep to this; identify line between posterior/superior EAC and inferior temporal line
     - Size 5 cutting burr and irrigation
     - Delineate tegmen and sigmoid sinus
     - Follow posterior canal wall
     - Through Korner's septum into antrum
     - Identify lateral semicircular canal
     - Identify short process incus (in the fossa incudes)
     - Posterior tympanotomy: 2 mm diamond burr
       - ■ Anteriorly CT, posteriorly CN VII

Canal Wall Down vs Up

	Canal Wall Down	*Canal Wall Up*
Advantages:	Low chance of residual disease Detection of recurrence easier	Physiological position of TM OCR maybe more stable, lengthier F/U periods
Disadvantages:	Lifelong water precautions Open cavity – long-term maintenance Shallow middle ear means difficult OCR	Higher risk of residual and recurrent disease Second stage/DWI MRI follow up required

Facial Nerve

1. Anatomy:
   - Innervates muscles of facial expression, carries fibres that convey taste from anterior 2/3 of tongue and supply pre-ganglionic parasympathetic fibres to head and neck ganglia

Nuclei	*Location*	*Function*
Motor nuclei	Pons	Muscles of facial expression, stapedius
Superior salivatory nuclei	Pons	Efferent to lacrimal, nasal, palatine, sublingual and submandibular glands
Nucleus solitarius	Medulla	Afferents from anterior 2/3 tongue
Sensory root	Nervus intermedius	

   - Segments (see Figure 3.6):
     - Intra-cranial segment: Brainstem to IAC
NI and motor root form common facial nerve
     - Intra-temporal segment:
       - ■ Meatal: Covered in meninges
8–10 mm
Fundus of IAM is divided vertically by Bill's bar and horizontally by Falciform crest; facial nerve is located antero-superiorly

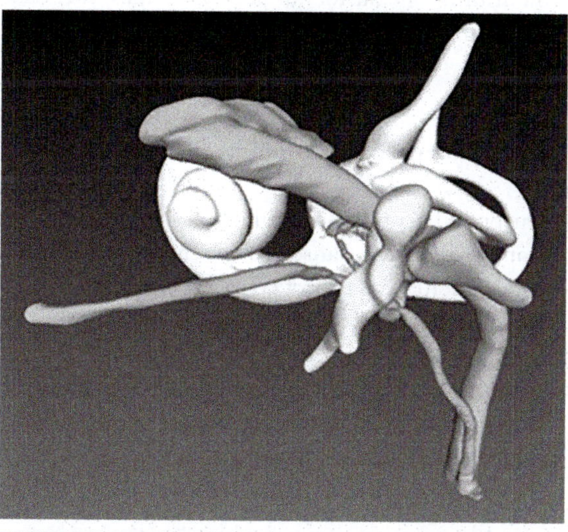

Figure 3.6 Computer generated render of the path of the facial nerve and chorda tympani in relation to the cochlea, semi-circular canals and ossicles.

- Labyrinthine: Narrowest segment (0.7 mm)
  4 mm from fundus to geniculate ganglion (superior to processus cochleariformis)
  GSPN exits at facial hiatus
- Tympanic: Below LSSC, above oval window
  Between first and second genu
  11 mm in length
- Mastoid segment: Branches to stapedius and chorda tympani
  13 mm in length from second genu to stylomastoid foramen

- Extra-temporal segment: At stylomastoid foramen
  - Posterior auricular nerve (motor)
  - Nerve to stylohyoid, posterior belly of digastric
  - Pes divides into temporozygomatic and cervicofacial branches

– Facial nerve surgical landmarks:
  - 1 cm deep and inferior to tragal pointer
  - Nerve trunk is posterior and lateral to styloid process. If encountered, dissection is too anterior and deep
  - 6–8 mm deep to tympanomastoid suture line
  - Antero-medial to insertion of posterior belly of digastric
  - Radiologically lies superficial to retromandibular vein (divides the parotid gland into superficial and deep lobes)

– Nerve fibre components:
  - Endoneurium: Surrounds individual axons
  - Perineurium: Surrounds nerve fasciculus, enclosing multiple axons
  - Epineurium: Outer layer consisting of vasa nervosum for nutrition

2. Injury:

Sunderland Nerve Injury Classification:

Class 1: Neuropraxia/compression injury
Class 2: Axonotmesis, axon transected but endoneurium intact (Wallerian degeneration): Can expect complete recovery
Class 3: Neurotmesis, transection of neural tube (axon, endoneurium): Usually leads to synkinesis
Class 4: Perineurium violated, only outer epineural sheath remains and distinguishes from class 5 injury: Surgery required
Class 5: Complete transection: Surgery required

– Nerve function tests:
  - NET (Nerve excitability test):
    - Lowest current to induce a twitch. Sides compared to deduce threshold difference. Electrode at SMF

- MST (Maximal stimulation test): Similar NET, but now maximal stimulation
  - Current required to create maximal amplitude of normal side and compared to paralysed side
- ENOG (Electroneurography): Best done at 3–21 days
  - Measures compound muscle action potentials (CMAP): Summation of APs of all functioning axons
  - CAP is proportional to number of intact axons
  - CN VII stimulated transcutaneously at stylomastoid foramen and sensory electrodes placed at branches of facial nerve
  - Percentage loss of function elicited, with >90% degeneration = poor prognosis
- EMG: Electromyography:
  - Complementary to above tests
  - Determines activity of muscle rather than nerve (hence myography)
  - useful for detecting denervation, or emerging reinnervation
  - Needle electrodes record spontaneous and voluntary motor unit action potentials

Facial Nerve Paralysis

1. Background:

Categories:

Idiopathic:	Bell's palsy (possibly re-activation of HSV-1 in geniculate ganglion)
Congenital:	Mobius (underdeveloped CN VI and VII), CULLP
Iatrogenic:	Middle ear (tympanic and vertical segments) or parotid surgery
Trauma:	Temporal bone fracture (RTA, assault) and birth trauma
Infective:	NOE, AOM, syphilis, Ramsay-Hunt, HIV, EBV, TB, Lyme's disease (other CNs affected)
Systemic:	Sarcoidosis, Wegener's, Amyloidosis, Melkersson-Rosenthal (facial oedema, CN VII palsy, cheilitis, fissured tongue)
Neurological:	MS, GBS, MG
Neoplasia:	Benign: Vestibular schwannoma, facial schwannoma, ossifying haemangioma, cholesteatoma, paraganglioma
Malignant:	Parotid, temporal bone, metastatic

2. History:
   - Age (also congenital)
   - Timing/onset (immediate or delayed following surgery) + complete vs incomplete
   - Trauma/recent surgery
   - Systemic symptoms and recent travel
   - Otalgia/hearing loss
   - PMH: Parotid cancers/RT, DM/Chemotherapy/HIV (MOE), syphilis
3. Examination:
   - Full neuro and CN examination (LMN palsy? acuity)
     - Facial nerve: Bell's phenomenon, paresis vs paralysis, eye closure
   - Head and neck examination:
     - Parotid/nodal masses
     - Ear examination: Vesicles and for AOM
4. Investigations:
   - None if typical Bell's palsy
   - FBC (anaemia of chronic disease), CRP, ESR, ACE/Ca (Sarcoidosis), VDRL (Syphilis), IgG/M (Borrelia Burgdorferi)
   - Audiometry (temporal bone trauma as baseline)
   - CT (temporal bone trauma, lesions, mastoiditis), MRI with gadolinium for neuromas/schwannomas or demyelinating disease
   - NCS: NET, MST, ENoG (evoked EMG, only for complete paralysis)
5. Management:

Facial Nerve Repair	
End-to-end (Neurorrhaphy): • Motor end plates intact (<12–18/12 of injury) • Recent injury (<3/7) • Where tension free closure is applicable	**Nerve crossover (Transposition)** • Distal segment intact, proximal missing (temp bone tumours) • Motor end plates intact • CN XII to VII via cable or end-to-side anastomosis OR • Cross-face (CN VII to VII) via cable graft
Cable grafting (Interposition): • Motor end plates intact. Tension free anastomosis not possible • Greater auricular or sural nerves • Provides resting muscle tone	

Static procedures (adjunct to enhance symmetry)	*Dynamic procedures (atrophic facial muscles or absent CN VII)*
• Facial, allograft, synthetic slings • Browlift • Canthoplasty (tightening of lower canthal tendon) • Rhytidoplasty (facelift) • Ocular: Tarsorrhaphy, weighted implants, botox (synkinesis)	• Temporalis muscle transposition (for eye) • Masseter muscle transposition (mouth) • Free nerve/muscle transposition (gracilis), innervated using a cable graft from CN VII to gracilis (side to side) and end to end with masseteric nerve (V3) or CN VII. Dual innervated flap

- MDT approach: ENT, ophthalmology, physiotherapy, plastics
- Conservative: In acute setting, tape eyes and consider early physiotherapy
- Medical:
  - Eye care: Viscotears and Lacri lube
  - Steroids in acute setting (delayed palsy following trauma or surgery) for complete palsy
    - Bell's: 10/7 of Prednisolone 50 mg (25 mg BD or 50 mg OD – as per Scottish Bell's Palsy Study)
  - Antibiotics in AOM or Lyme's. Antivirals in Ramsay-Hunt (limited evidence)

6. Evidence:
   - See Sullivan et al. Early treatment with Prednisolone or Aciclovir in Bell's Palsy. NEJM 2007; 357(16):1598–1607
     - At 9/12, Prednisolone cohort 94% recovery vs 81% with no intervention
   - See Monsanto et al. Treatment and Prognosis of Facial Palsy on Ramsay Hunt Syndrome. Int Arch Otolaryngology 2016; 20(4): 394–400:
     - 2/3 achieve full/grade II recovery following steroids + Aciclovir
   - Cochrane (2008): Use of antivirals in Ramsay-Hunt syndrome:
     - One low-powered study, showing no benefit. Consider risk vs benefit

House-Brackmann Scale

Grade Description	Characteristics
I:	Normal
II:	Slight: Mild weakness
III:	Moderate: Facial asymmetry and weakness but eye closes
IV:	Moderately severe: Total facial asymmetry and weakness with incomplete closure of the eye
V:	Severe: Barely detectable movement
VI:	Total: No facial function

Benign Paroxysmal Positional Vertigo

1. Background:
   - Most common cause of vertigo in elderly
   - Posterior canal > lateral canal > superior canal
   - Causes: Spontaneous (1/3 idiopathic), post-viral (labyrinthitis), post-trauma
     - May co-exist with other pathology: Meniere's, Vit D deficiency
   - Mechanism:
     - Canal lithiasis: Otoconia within endolymph of SSC, which then displace cupula through inertia and result in vertigo
     - Cupulolithiasis: Otoconia adhere to cupula of SSC, which then becomes sensitive to gravity
2. History:
   - Brief episodes of vertigo on head movement lasting sec to min, normal in between
   - Otology symptoms: Hearing loss, infections, tinnitus, autophony, Tulio's phenomenon to rule out other causes
   - Ask: Falls and impact on quality of life, surgery in past
   - PMH: Trauma, Vit D levels, previous surgery (perilymph fistula), otosclerosis, Meniere's, migraine
   - FH: Hearing loss
   - Rule out central vertebrobasilar insufficiency: (Ds) dysarthria, dysphagia, dysesthesia, diplopia
3. Examination:
   - Otoscopy
   - Cranial nerve examination
   - Eyes:
     - Saccadic system: Shifting of gaze from one object to another:
       - ■ Over/undershoot, delay or slow movement = brainstem/cerebellar pathology. NB: Small undershoot (hypometric saccades) are normal
     - Smooth pursuit: Maintain gaze on mobile object:
       - ■ Bilateral impairment: Drug induced (psychotropic and alcohol), age, fatigue, CNS/cerebellar
     - Head impulse test: Tests VOR. With fast thrust, eyes should remain focused on object
       - ■ Corrective saccade seen in peripheral pathology
     - Romberg's test: Assessment of proprioception, cerebellum, vestibular system and vision, positive if unsteady with eyes closed
     - Unterberger's test: Assessment of peripheral vestibular lesion, rotation to affected side

- Nystagmus: Frenzel goggles (magnifying glass goggles with light, eliminate fixation)
  - ■ Direction of nystagmus is described by direction of fast movements of eyes
  - ■ Vertical nystagmus is central in origin
  - ■ Alexander's laws:
    - o Fast phase is in opposite direction of endolymph flow
    - o Nystagmus is in the plane of SCC stimulated
    - o Amplitude is largest when looking in direction of fast phase
- Dix-Hallpike test: Assessment of posterior canal BPPV
  - ■ Positive if geotropic rotational nystagmus with latency of several sec towards affected ear
  - ■ In posterior canal BPPV, it will be rotatory with an upbeat component
  - ■ Lateral canal: Roll test

4. Investigations:
   - PTA, tympanometry ± vestibular function tests if indicated
   - Vitamin D levels if recurrent
   - MRI only for hearing loss, atypical nystagmus, central signs or persistent symptoms
5. Management:
   - Multi-disciplinary approach
   - Conservative: Vestibular rehabilitation, Brandt-Daroff exercises, Epley for posterior, Semont (if Epley fails or C-spine issues), BBQ roll or Gufoni for lateral canal
   - Medical: Not routinely used, but can consider anti-emetics for debilitating symptoms, Vitamin D
   - Surgical: Posterior canal occlusion/obliteration or vestibular neurectomy (poor hearing outcomes)

Characteristics of central vs peripheral nystagmus

	Central Nystagmus	*Peripheral Nystagmus*
Fatigue	No	Yes
Severity	Low	Debilitating
Fixation	No effect	Suppressed
Direction	Multiple	Horizontal (except BPPV which can have torsional/vertical components)
Conjugate	±	Yes

Ménière's Disease

1. Background:
   - Theories:
     - Endolymphatic hydrops due to:
       - Fluid build-up from saccin overproduction
       - Fibrosis of endolymphatic duct/sac resulting in impaired absorption/overdistension of membranous labyrinth
       - Autoimmune mechanisms
       - Distension of membranous labyrinth > microtears > mix of endolymph and perilymph resulting in hair cell damage
   - Usually unilateral, bilateral in 20%, genetic component, M = F, fourth to sixth decade, 60–80% remission naturally
   - Triad of: Vertigo, fluctuating SNHL, tinnitus (± aural fullness)
   - Initially reversible hearing loss, but eventually permanent (mainly low, but eventually all frequencies)
   - Variations:
     - Cochlear hydrops: No vertiginous features
     - Vestibular hydrops: No otological features (tinnitus or hearing loss; consider vestibular migraine)
     - Lermoyez syndrome: Symptoms relieved by vertigo, i.e. the tinnitus, fullness and hearing loss
     - Tumarkin crisis: Drop attack

International Classification of Vestibular Disorders (Lopez-Escamez et al. 2015)*	
Definite	*Probable*
≥2 spontaneous episodes of vertigo, each lasting 20 min to 12 hrs PTA confirmed low-mid frequency SNHL, before/during/after episode (at least 30 dB HL worse in affected ear at 2 contiguous frequencies <2 kHz) Fluctuating symptoms (aural fullness, tinnitus, hearing loss) within 24 hrs of vertigo episode No other vestibular diagnosis likely	Spontaneous vestibular symptoms (vertigo or dizziness) lasting 20 min to 24 hrs associated with: Fluctuating symptoms (aural fullness, tinnitus, hearing loss) No other vestibular diagnosis likely

Note:

*Lopez-Escamez JA et al. Diagnostic criteria for Menière's disease. JVR 2015; 25(1): 1–7.

2. History:
   - Vertigo lasting minutes to hours

   - Onset and duration of symptoms, pattern of episode, hearing loss (worse during attacks), otalgia, otorrhoea
   - Between attacks? Frequency and severity, triggers. Drop attacks (driving still? Warning symptoms?)
   - Medications tried
   - Migraine (DDx): History of migraines, personal and family, photophobia during attacks
3. Examination:
   - Otoscopy
   - Peripheral vestibulopathy: Romberg's/Unterberger's, head thrust
   - Dix Hallpike
   - Eyes to rule out central causes: Smooth pursuit, saccades, nystagmus
4. Investigations:
   - PTA: May demonstrate low-frequency SNHL, or fluctuation between tests at different times
   - Vestibular function tests: Hypofunction effected side (not needed unless doing ablative treatment)
   - Calorics: Tests LSSC only
     - Endolymph moving towards ampulla (ampullopetal) causes excitation in LSSC
     - Eye movement follows the flow of endolymph, with fast phase/nystagmus in opposite direction
     - Warm fluid causes ampullopetal movement of endolymph, and cold the opposite
     - COWS: Cold Opposite Warm Same dictates direction of fast phase of nystagmus
     - Canal paresis: Reduced or absent response compared to contralateral side due to peripheral lesion
       - Values above 25% deemed significant
   - ECoG: SP:AP ratio > 0.4
   - VEMPs: Increased threshold, reduced amplitude
   - MRI IAM: In the event of unilateral SNHL
   - Glycerol dehydration test/mannitol improves symptoms within 30–60 min
5. Management:
   - If unprovoked episodes with no warning, must advise to discontinue driving and inform DVLA
   - Conservative:
     - Dietary/lifestyle: <1.5 g salt intake, reduce alcohol/caffeine, stress avoidance, support group, kg loss
     - Hearing aid
     - Tinnitus retraining therapy

- Medical:
  - Bendroflumethiazide 1.25 mg increments: Controversial with limited evidence
  - Betahistine: Low-level evidence to suggest improvement in middle ear blood flow, up to 32 mg TDS
  - Prochlorperazine during acute attacks
  - Intra-tympanic steroid (hearing sparing, 90% response, dexamethasone 3.3 mg/mL or methylprednisolone 62.5 mg/mL)
  - Vestibulo Ablative gentamicin (if unilateral with little audiological reserve, 40 mg/mL, 5–10% risk hearing loss, 85% vertigo control). One dose 2-weeks apart
    - Middle ear volume 1.5–2.0 mL
- Surgical:
  - Grommet (anecdotal)
  - Endolymphatic sac surgery: Bony decompression or shunt (Donaldson's line)
  - Vestibular nerve section via craniotomy, aims to preserve hearing
  - Labyrinthectomy if no aidable hearing remaining. Not if poor vestibular function in contra-lateral ear

6. Differential diagnosis
   - BPPV
   - Acute labyrinthitis/neuronitis
   - Migrainous vertigo
   - Ménière's syndrome: Cogan's, syphilis, trauma
   - Stroke
   - Multiple sclerosis
   - Variants:
     - Lermoyez variant: Hearing loss and tinnitus precede episode of vertigo by weeks, hearing improves with attack
     - Cochlear hydrops: No vestibular symptoms
     - Vestibular hydrops: No cochlear symptoms
7. Evidence:
   - Cochrane database (2001): Use of betahistine in Meniere's disease
     - Insufficient evidence
   - BEMED trial, BMJ (2016): Efficacy and safety of betahistine treatment in patients with Meniere's disease: Primary results of a long term, multicentre, double blind, randomised, placebo controlled, dose defining trial (BEMED trial)
     - Limited evidence
   - Cochrane database (2011): Intratympanic steroids for Meniere's disease or syndrome
     - Statistically significant reduction in symptoms at 24 months

  - Cochrane database (2018): Dietary changes in the treatment of Meniere's disease or syndrome
    - Insufficient evidence

Superior Semicircular Canal Dehiscence Syndrome

1. Background:
   - First described by Lloyd B Minor in 1998
   - F > M
   - Reduction or absence of bone overlying superior semi-circular canal that allows inner ear fluid to be displaced by sound or pressure stimuli – third window hypothesis
     - Air conducted sound dissipates through third window, resulting in increased AC thresholds
     - BC reduced thresholds: i.e. increased sensitivity to bone conducted sound due to reduced impedance of the third window allowing sound to enter perilymph through the labyrinth, resulting in better hearing thresholds
   - Aetiology: Trauma, middle fossa surgery, raised CSF pressure, congenital dehiscence
2. History:
   - Hearing loss
   - BC hypersensitivity
   - Vertigo
   - Tinnitus: Pulsatile
   - Aural fullness
   - Autophony: Speech, heartbeat, eye movements, footsteps (BC hypersensitivity)
   - Tullio phenomenon: Vertigo to loud noise
   - Dizziness on straining
   - Hennebert's sign: Pressure induced vertigo or nystagmus (insufflate EAC)
3. Examination:
   - Otoscopy: Usually normal
   - Tests:
     - Fistula test: Positive
     - Valsalva test: Positive
     - Tulio's phenomenon: Positive
     - Nystagmus is usually in the plane of the SSC, and if in any other plane, re-consider diagnosis
     - Low-frequency tuning fork on ankle heard in affected ear
4. Investigations:
   - Audiometry: Low-frequency CHL (pseudo ABG)

   - Stapedial reflexes: Normal
   - cVEMP: Ipsilateral contraction of SCM to sound (reduced thresholds and raised amplitude)
   - Electrocochleaography: Elevated SP/AP ratio
   - HRCT (0.5 mm slice) of temporal bones reconstruction on Poschl's and Stenvers planes
5. Management:
   - Conservative:
     - Vestibular rehabilitation
     - Tinnitus retraining therapy
     - Air conduction aids
   - Medical:
     - Vestibular sedatives (short-term use only)
   - Surgical:
     - Re-surfacing or plugging of the SSC
       - Middle cranial fossa vs trans-mastoid
6. Differential diagnoses:
   - Otosclerosis
   - Ménière's disease
   - Perilymph fistula
   - Other third window

Causes of Tulio phenomenon

- Superior semicircular canal dehiscence
- Posterior semicircular canal dehiscence
- Cholesteatoma leading to semicircular canal erosion
- Perilymph fistula
- Ménière's disease
- Syphilis (as per original description by Prof Pietro Tullio)
- Trauma
- Iatrogenic: Stapedectomy, tympanomastoidectomy

Necrotising Otitis Externa/Malignant Otitis Externa

1. Background:
   - Most commonly pseudomonas (Gram-positive rod), proteus, staphylococcus
   - Aspergillus most common fungal (also seen in HIV patients)
   - Pseudomonas has mortality of 40–60% throughout hospital medicine
   - Can result in skull base osteomyelitis through fissures of Santorini (breaks in hyaline cartilage) or foramen of Huschke (dehiscence in tympanic ring)

2. History:
   - Otalgia+++
   - Otitis externa/discharge
   - Intractable pain, trismus (TMJ and masseteric space), and worse nocturnally
   - PMH:
     - DM: Most common, HIV, chemotherapy, radiotherapy, other immunosuppression
   - DH: DMARDs, steroids etc.
3. Examination:
   - Otological examination: Discharge, granulation tissue/polyp in osseo-cartilaginous junction, with exposed bone
   - Cranial nerve examination: Palsies of VII but also involving hypoglossal canal (XI) and jugular foramen (IX, X, XI) (neurotoxin release or mass effect from inflammatory tissue)
     - Associated with poorer outcome
4. Investigations:
   - Surgical: Biopsy of polyp/granulation tissue to rule out underlying SCC
   - Biochemistry/haematology: FBC, U&E's, CRP, ESR (0–20), HbA1c, glucose
   - Radiology:
     - CT first line for erosive changes: Mastoid, ear canal, TMJ, foramina
     - MRI for soft tissue changes and marrow oedema
     - Rare: Tc-99m for active disease (high osteoblastic activity)
     - Rare: Gd-67 for monitoring (nuclear medicine)
     - Rare: Indium-111 WCC scan for monitoring (nuclear medicine)
5. Management:
   - See ENT-UK Guidelines for more detail
   - MDT involvement: ENT, microbiology, infectious diseases, neuroradiology, endocrinology
   - Conservative:
     - Microsuction
     - Eye care if facial palsy
   - Medical: Dependent on severity
     - Medical optimisation (glycaemic control, HbA1c)
     - IV antibiotics
       - Based on local antimicrobial policies, usually through long line
       - IV 6 weeks, PO 6 weeks (Meropenem and Piperacillin/Tazobactam (Tazocin) acceptable regimes but depends on local sensitivities and policy)
     - In mild cases, can consider outpatient PO Ciprofloxacin, but must be aware of risk of C. Diff in elderly patients
   - Surgical: EUA + biopsy to rule out malignancy (often performed under LA in outpatients)

6. Differential diagnoses:
   - Malignancy (SCC)
   - Osteoradionecrosis
   - Granulomatosis with Polyangiitis (GPA – previously called Wegener's Granulomatosis)
   - Paget's/fibrous dysplasia

Otosclerosis

1. Background:
   - Autosomal dominant with incomplete penetrance. 70% bilateral
   - Metabolic disorder of bone (affects all three layers of otic capsule and ossicles)
   - Phases:
     - Lytic: Increased osteoclastic activity leads to resorption and fibrotic spaces
     - Bony: Increased osteoblastic activity in fibrotic spaces leads to deposition of immature bone
     - Re-modelling: Cycling leads to sclerotic bone deposition
   - Pathophysiology
     - 10% Caucasians have histology dx but only <1% symptomatic
     - Measles history/SERPINF1 gene
     - Accelerated by pregnancy (debatable but commonly claimed), female > male
     - Fixation secondary to annular ligament calcification or footplate involvement (80% fissula ante fenestram)
   - Hearing loss of 1 dB (ABG per annum)
   - Target ABG < 10 dB
2. History:
   - Age of onset
   - Typically progressive. May be unilateral/bilateral. Typically CHL but may progress to mixed/SNHL in cochlear OS
   - Tinnitus is a feature of 75–80% of otosclerosis patients
   - Vertigo uncommon
   - Paracusis Willisii: CHL causes reduction of background noise and people raise their voices, hence hearing may improve in busy environments
   - PMH: Pregnancy and deterioration in symptoms (accelerated by Oestrogen)
   - FH: Hearing loss or surgery
3. Examination:
   - Otoscopy usually normal
     - Schwartz's sign: Red/blue hue over promontory and oval window niche due to active otosclerosis with rich vascular supply

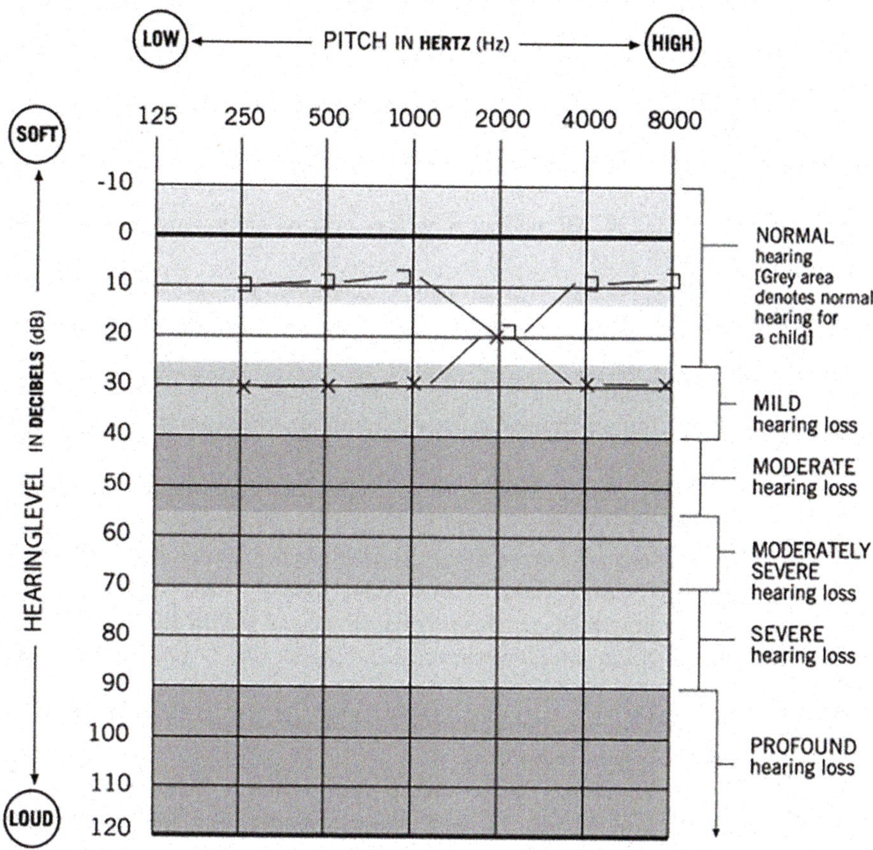

Figure 3.7 Pure tone audiogram showing air and bone conduction thresholds for the left ear with Carhart's Notch at 2kHz. The most likely cause for this would be otosclerosis, though any cause of a conductive hearing loss can cause Carhart's Notch.

- Reversal of tuning fork test (Rinne negative to positive when using 512 then 1024 Hz): Ensures large ABG

4. Investigations:
   - Audiometry (see Figure 3.7): Carhart's notch: Artefactual dip in bone conduction at 2 kHz in CHL. Improves on correction of conductive loss
     - 2 kHz is resonance frequency at which ossicles transmit sound most efficiently
   - Tympanometry: Type As (stiff, low compliance)
   - Stapedial reflexes (absent in otosclerosis)
   - Speech audiometry: Cochlear otosclerosis if SDS <60% (likely poor surgical candidate), if presented at least 40 dB SL

- CT: Alternative diagnosis suspected, for middle ear anatomy. Halo sign around cochlea (advanced disease/cochlear otosclerosis)

5. Management:
   - Conservative (first line, especially if family planning): Air conduction aid first line, consider bone conduction aid (ABG)
   - Medical:
     - Fluoride (20–40 mg/day) stabilises hearing by slowing active disease – evidence low
     - Bisphosphonates (risedronate, zoledronate) may slow cochlear otosclerosis
   - Surgical:
     - Stapedectomy
       - 0.7 mm drill used, with a 0.6 mm prosthesis (may also use KTP laser)
       - CHL >15 dB ABG, with good speech discrimination >60%(similar to BAHA criteria)
       - Risks: Facial nerve <1%, taste disturbance, dead ear (0.5–1%), CT injury, displacement, tinnitus, vertigo, prosthesis displacement
       - Around 80% get closure of air bone gap within 10 dB
       - Revision cases lower success and higher risk 7× profound hearing loss
       - Operate on poorer hearing ear first (second after 6–12/12)
       - Contraindications:
         - Absolute: Active otosclerosis, cochlear otosclerosis, active CSOM/OE, Meniere's disease, malleus ankylosis
         - Relative: Only hearing ear, aberrant facial nerve/stapedial artery (continue if <50% of footplate, or cauterize if small), pre-op speech discrimination <60%
       - Other considerations:
         - Biscuit footplate: Microdrill and prosthesis
         - Floating footplate: Risk of depressing into vestibule. Abort, allow to re-fix and repeat
6. Differential diagnoses:
   - Ossicular fixation/discontinuity, TS
   - Malleus head fixation
   - Poorly masked audiogram
   - Glue ear
   - Superior canal dehiscence
   - Paget's disease, fibrous dysplasia or osteogenesis imperfecta
7. Evidence:
   - Hentschel et al. Limited evidence for the effect of sodium fluoride on deterioration of hearing loss in patients with otosclerosis: a systematic review of the literature. Otol Neurotol 2014; 35(6): 1052–1057

- Weak evidence of reduction in hearing loss compared to placebo – one study only
- Low-level evidence (case series) advocating use of bisphosphonates

Perilymph gusher management:

- Seal (vein patch/fascia)
- Place prosthesis
- Pack gelfoam

Ear Canal Exostosis and Osteomas

1. Background:
   - Exostoses:
     - Unknown aetiology although association with cold water or air exposure (surfer's ear)
     - Usually seen in medial canal wall
     - Unilateral or bilateral
     - Single or multiple
     - More sessile (osseo-cartilaginous junction)
   - Osteoma:
     - True neoplastic growth: Smooth, pedunculated
     - Symptomatic if occlusive in nature
     - Usually solitary lesion
     - Hard/firm lesions (bone-bone junction (Gardner's syndrome)
     - Can be genetic: Associated with APC gene mutation and colonic polyps
2. History:
   - Risk factors for development (exostoses) i.e. cold water exposure
   - Ear symptoms:
     - Hearing loss
     - Recurrent infections
     - Wax impaction
   - Impact on social or work life/ability to wear HAs if required
3. Examination:
   - Otoscopy
     - Evaluate lesions:
       - Positioning (medial vs lateral)
       - Base (broad vs pedunculated)
       - Quantity (single vs multiple)

    - Otitis externa/wax impaction
  - Facial nerve
4. Investigations:
   - Swab for MC&S
   - Audiometry (assess for CHL)
   - CT
5. Management:
   - Conservative: If asymptomatic (usually osteomas)
   - Medical:
     - Sodium bicarbonate for impacted wax
     - Topical steroid/antibiotics for otitis externa
   - Surgical:
     - Canalplasty for obstructive and symptomatic cases
     - Osteomas can usually be removed endoscopically or using drill
     - Post-aural approach usually reserved for multiple exostosis

Characteristics of exostosis vs osteomas

Exostosis	*Osteoma*
No fibrovascular channels	Marrow spaces and fibrovascular channels (tumour, so angiogenesis occurs)
Medial aspect of EAC/ osseocartilaginous junction	Found on tympanosquamous and tympanomastoid suture lines (bony junctions)
Bilateral, broad base	Unilateral, pedunculated
Cold water exposure association	True neoplastic growth
Canalplasty if symptomatic using endoscopic approach	Post-aural or permeatal approach

Gardner's syndrome ("Familial adenomatous polyposis"):

- Autosomal dominant, present in third decade
- APC gene chromosome 5q22
- Osteomas
- Colonic polyps (polyps progress to colorectal cancer)
- Epidermoid cysts
- Supernumerary teeth
- Papillary thyroid Ca

Eustachian Tube Dysfunction and Patulous Eustachian Tube

1. Background:
   - Eustachian tube (ET) problems are common, sometimes difficult to diagnose and often difficult to improve
   - The ET has three main functions: (i) pressure equalisation and ventilation of the middle ear, (ii) mucociliary clearance of middle ear secretions and (iii) protection of the middle ear from sounds, pathogens and secretions from the nasopharynx
   - May be acute (<3 months) or chronic (>3 months)
   - The three main subtypes of ETD are (i) dilatory ETD (typically functional obstruction, muscular failure or anatomical obstruction), (ii) barochallenge induced ETD and (iii) patulous ETD
   - Patulous eustachian tube (PET) describes a widely open ET causing increased air transfer into ME typical symptoms are: Autophony, aerophony, aural fullness
2. History:
   - Commonly complains about popping/clicking (often physiological), aural fullness, discomfort/pain, "under water" sensation, muffled hearing
   - PET worse as day goes on or after exercise
   - Commonly worse when exposed to baro-challenge (diving/flying)
   - PET: Weight loss, RT, habitual sniffing
   - Neurological problems: CVA, Myasthenia gravis
   - Iatrogenic to TVP as innervated by V3 (opens ET on swallowing/yawning)
3. Examination:
   - PET on FNE
   - Otoscopic mobility of TM on breathing (sign of PET)
   - PET autophony better on lying down
4. Investigations:
   - Typically, none in UK but variety of tympanometry tests can be performed
5. Management:
   - Conservative
   - Medical: PET
     - Topical oestrogen drops: Increase torus swelling
     - Douching with distilled water
     - Obstructive: Steroid nasal sprays (limited if any benefit)
   - Surgical:
     - Grommet (both obstructive and PET)
     - Inject hyaluronic acid into Eustachian cushion (PET)
     - Pack ET (fat, gelfoam), cartilage graft

Vestibular Schwannoma

1. Background:
   - Tumour of Schwann cells of vestibular nerve, and most common lesion in CPA (adults) – 80% of tumours at CPA and 8% of all intracranial tumours. T1/T2 hypointense but bright on T1 with contrast
   - One-third will grow in 1–3 yrs, half will grow by 5 yrs; growth in first yearr predicts further tumour growth; average growth rate of 1 mm/year (Paldor I et al. Growth rate of vestibular schwannoma. J Clin Neurosci. 2016; 32: 1–8)
   - <1% malignant transformation
   - Sporadic in 95%, genetic in 5% (consider if <30 yrs)
   - Phases of growth:
     - Otological phase: Progressive or sudden SNHL + tinnitus. Vertigo if increased growth (bleed). Hitzelberger's sign
     - Neurological phase (extension into CPA): Headaches, cranial nerve compression, ataxia, rare: Diplopia (CN6 palsy), hoarseness and dysphagia (CN9/10)
     - Terminal phase: Raised ICP/GCS, failing vision/papilloedema
2. History:
   - Most commonly present with asymmetric SNHL/sudden HL (10%), tinnitus and vertigo
   - Dependent on size of tumour and location
   - Cranial nerve symptoms include CNV paraesthesia
3. Examination:
   - Full otological examination:
   - Cranial nerve examination:
     - Facial nerve involvement: Palsy, Hitzelberger sign (hypoesthesia of posterior meatal wall), reduced lacrimation (Schirmer's test), loss of taste
   - Cerebellar examination: Gait, hypotonia, intention tremor, nystagmus, in later stages Brun's nystagmus
4. Investigations:
   - Audiometry:
     - Rollover phenomenon: Reduction in word recognition score (speech recognition score) with increasing intensity
     - Phonemic regression: Disproportionate speech recognition when compared to pure tone thresholds
     - Tone decay/fatigue: Decreased auditory perception with sustained signal stimulus – retro-cochlear pathology
   - ABR: Interaural latency on wave V (sensitive only to tumours >1.5 cm), or increased I–V latency

- Imaging:
  - CT may show widening of IAC, and bone resorption (unlike hyperostosis in meningioma)
  - MRI: Iso/hypo-intense on T1, T2. Hyperintense on Ga contrast, arising from IAC, with cystic component

5. Management:
   - Multi-disciplinary approach
   - Conservative: If <20 mm in size, or growth of <1 mm/year
     - Most commonly adopted:
       - 6 monthly scans (year 1), yearly (years 2, 3, 4), then every other year, then every 3 yrs if no growth
       - Potentially discharge if no growth for 5 yrs (probability of growth <5%) (Sethi et al. The conditional probability of vestibular schwannoma growth at different time points after initial stability on an observational protocol. Otol Neurotol. 2020; 41(2): 250–257)
   - Medical: If <25 mm (due to rebound oedema) + growing >2 mm/year
     - Avastin: May arrest tumour progression/hearing loss in select NF2 patients, serious adverse events
     - Radiotherapy: Aims to stabilise size, now used often
       - Stereotactic: Gamma knife surgery, cyberknife or fractionated
   - Surgical:
     - Translabyrinthine:
       - Highest facial nerve preservation, wide view, minimal brain retraction
       - Non-hearing preservation surgery
     - Middle fossa:
       - Landmarks: GSPN, arcuate eminence and MMA
       - Small intra-canalicular tumours (small CPA component <1 cm in size), with good hearing preservation
       - Some risk of epilepsy due to temporal lobe retraction (requires anti-epileptics, thus cannot drive for 12 months in UK), facial nerve injury rates higher
     - Retrosigmoid:
       - Good hearing preservation, wide view (any sized tumour), good facial nerve preservation
       - Cerebellar retraction
       - Largest tumours
     - Complications: GA, CSF leak, meningitis, SIADH + above specific to procedure
6. Differential diagnoses:
   - Meningeal pathology: Meningioma: More homogenous, calcified and dural tail, arachnoid cyst (thin walled with CSF) and metastasis (breast, renal, prostate, thyroid, kidney, lung)

  - CNS pathology: CN VII schwannoma (enlarged fallopian canal) or malignant nerve sheath tumour
  - Skull base pathology: Chordoma, chondrosarcoma and cholesterol granuloma
  - Cisterns (subarachnoid space): Epidermoid cyst (congenital cholesteatoma of CPA), arachnoid cyst and lipoma

Neurofibromatosis (NF2)

1. Background:
   - NF1 (von Recklinghausen):
     - Neurofibromin mutation on chromosome 17
     - Increased risk of sarcomas, avoid radiotherapy
     - Neurofibroma types:
       - Cutaneous
       - Subcutaneous
       - Nodule plexiform (along clusters of nerve roots as nodular suggests)
       - Diffuse plexiform (congenital along large segments of nerves): Highest risk of malignancy
     - Vestibular schwannoma 5%
   - NF2:
     - Suspect in any child under the age of 30 with a VS
     - Autosomal dominant, but 50% have no family history
     - Mutation on NF2 gene on long arm of chromosome 22, which encodes for Merlin protein (tumour suppressor)
     - Subcapsular cataracts diagnostic
     - Bilateral VS's diagnostic, by age 30 yrs

Diagnostic Criteria (NIH Criteria plus (additional) Manchester Criteria)

Bilateral vestibular schwannomas or family history of NF2 plus

- Unilateral VS or
- Any two of:
  - meningioma
  - glioma
  - neurofibroma
  - schwannoma
  - posterior subcapsular lenticular opacities

Additional criteria

- Unilateral VS plus any two of
  - meningioma
  - glioma
  - neurofibroma
  - schwannoma
  - posterior subcapsular lenticular opacities

or

- Multiple meningiomas (two or more) plus
  - Unilateral VS or any two of:
    - glioma
    - neurofibroma
    - schwannoma
    - cataract

   - NF2 hearing rehabilitation options:
     - If non-serviceable hearing and intact cochlear nerves: Cochlear implantation
     - If non-serviceable hearing and cochlear nerve loss: Brainstem implant
2. History: See "Vestibular Schwannoma":
   - If genetic component, patients will have a history of presentation commonly between 18 and 24 yrs of age
3. Examination:
   - Full otological examination
   - Cranial nerve examination
     - Hitzelberger sign: Reduced sensation conchal bowl and floor of EAC due to lesion within IAC
     - Facial hypoesthesia, Absent corneal reflex
     - Facial nerve exam (can be associated with facial nerve schwannomas)
   - Cerebellar examination
4. Management: See vestibular schwannoma handout:
   - MDT approach at specialist NF2 unit
   - May include Avastin (Bevacizumab) an inhibitor of Vascular Endothelial Growth Factor-A (VEGF-A). Typically if growning 3mm/year or more
5. Investigations:
   - Audiological investigation:
     - Include ABR
   - Ophthalmology assessment
   - Dermatological assessment for evaluation of cutaneous lesions
   - Genetic testing and family counselling

- Imaging:
  - MRI head/spine in initial instance
    - For surveillance: From 10 yrs of age annually
6. Differential diagnoses:
   - See "Vestibular Schwannoma"

Paraganglioma

1. Background:
   - Benign neuroendocrine tumours, arising from neural crest cells (ectodermal layer), which migrate and form peripheral nervous system
   - 90% adrenal (pheochromocytoma in 20–40%), 10% extra-adrenal, of which 85% abdominal, and 3% head and neck; "Rule of 10%" (10% metastatic, 10% familial, 10% recurring, 10% extra-adrenal, 10% paediatric)
   - F>M, fifth decade, 2 per million, 1–3% associated with paraneoplastic syndrome
   - WHO classification according to location: Carotid body > jugulare > tympanicum > vagal
   - Supplied by ascending pharyngeal artery. Carotid body supplied by the carotid sinus nerve (CN IX)
   - Related to SDH complex: SDH-B poor prognosis, SDH-D Dad "parent-of-origin" effect
     - Malignancy rate <5% – SDH-B mutation: Present with nodal metastasis
2. History: Depends on suspected tumour site
   - Jugular/tympanic: Pulsatile tinnitus, hearing loss (conductive), vertigo implies invasion into labyrinth. CN palsy IV–XII
   - Carotid: Painless neck mass, dysphagia, CN palsies and Horner's syndrome
   - Vagal: Dysphagia, dysphonia, pain, cough, aspiration
   - FH: Genetic component
3. Examination: Depends on tumour site
   - Full head and neck examination for palpable masses
     - Aquino's sign: Reduction in pulsation with carotid artery compression
     - Fontaine sign: Carotid mass moves laterally and not vertically
   - Otoscopy, and audiometry/tympanometry to assess for conductive deficit
     - Rising sun sign on otoscopy
     - Brown's sign: Blanching with positive pressure on TM
4. Investigations:
   - CT temporal bones may demonstrate bony erosion (moth-eaten appearance)
     - Phelp's sign = Erosion of caroticojugular spine between carotid canal and jugular fossa
   - MRI/A: Salt and pepper appearance on T2, in vascular masses with focus of haemorrhage
   - 4-vessel-angiography

    - Lyre's sign: Splaying of the internal and external carotid arteries due to carotid body or vagal paraganglioma
  - FDG-PET to assess for synchronous tumours: ONLY if plasma catecholamines are raised as well as positive genetics
  - USS ± FNAC (if non-glomus pathology)
  - Urinary catecholamines (VMA, normetanephrine), plasma metanephrines if flushing, headaches, palpitations
  - Whole body MRI to r/o other synchronous tumours
5. Management:
  - Skull base MDT and genetic screening
  - Conservative: For asymptomatic small tumours and those unfit for medical/surgical intervention
  - Medical: EBRT for multiple/larger tumours, recurrence or incomplete resection. Stereotactic for smaller tumours
  - Surgical: Particularly if CN palsies and may warrant pre-op embolisation. Subtotal resection if too large
    - Lateral skull base/infra-temporal fossa approach for larger tumours with poor access
6. Differential diagnoses:
  - Glue ear
  - Haemotympanum
  - Otosclerosis (Schwartz sign)
  - Aberrant carotid artery/high riding jugular bulb/persistent stapedial artery

Fisch classification:

A:	Middle ear only	
B:	Tympanomastoid	
C:	Labyrinthine/petrous involvement	
	C1	Carotid foramen
	C2	Vertical aspect of carotid canal
	C3	Horizontal aspect of carotid canal
	C4	Foramen lacerum
D:	Intracranial	
	DI	Extradural extension (1 and 2 either <2 cm or >2 cm)
	DII	Intradural extension (1 and 2 either <2 cm or >2 cm)

Shamblin classification: Carotid involvement, and surgical resectability

I:	Easily localised and resected
II:	Adherent to nearby vessels
III:	Encasing carotids

Glassock-Jackson classification: Middle ear and mastoid

I: Promontory
II: Middle ear
III: Middle ear and mastoid
IV: Through TM into EAC

Temporal Bone Trauma

1. Background:
   - Classification:
     - Otic capsule involvement: This is the preferred classification method as clinically relevant
       - Otic capsule sparing (temporoparietal trauma):
         - Conductive hearing loss
         - Ossicular discontinuity or haemotympanum (involvement of middle ear cleft)
         - Canal laceration may be present with bleeding
       - Otic capsule involvement (occipital trauma): Foramen magnum across petrous bone to capsule
         - Predictive of serious complications as compared to otic sparing
         - SNHL due to damage to cochlea and vestibular structures (7–25× increased risk)
         - Higher rates of CN VII palsy (50%) (2–5× increased risk)
         - CSF (4–8× increased risk) and intra-cranial complications
     - Fracture path: Often mixed
       - Longitudinal (80%): Squamous portion, medially along EAC, roof of middle ear into petrous apex
       - Transverse (20%)
   - Fractures follow path of least resistance, so CN foramina usually involved
   - Facial palsy 7% (usually peri-geniculate ganglion region)/
   - Hearing loss often immediate
     - SNHL: Disruption of membranous labyrinth, avulsion of cochlear nerve, disruption of cochlear blood supply, cochlear haemorrhage or perilymph fistula
     - Conductive due to dislocation of ISJ and stapes crura fracture
   - Tinnitus is not a prognostic indicator
2. History:
   - Mechanism of injury: RTA, assault
   - Bleeding/otorrhoea/rhinorrhoea, hearing loss, vertigo (often not possible to assess if intubated at scene)

- Neurological status: Confusion, fluctuating, LOC, emesis
- Immediate or delayed CN VII palsy

3. Examination:
   - Initially using ATLS assessment: CABCD (trauma team primary then secondary survey)
   - Full neurological examination:
     - GCS (raised ICP from haemorrhage)
     - CN assessment, particularly CN VII (delayed or immediate)
   - Otoscopy/rhinoscopy:
     - Ear canal laceration, bleeding, haemotympanum, perforation, CSF otorrhoea (beta-2-transferrin)
     - Tuning fork tests at bedside if conscious patient
     - Battle's sign: Mastoid ecchymosis along distribution of posterior auricular artery
4. Investigations:
   - Audiometry: SNHL, CHL, ossicular chain discontinuity (avoid tympanometry as can cause pneumocephalus)
   - Stapedial reflexes (CN VII injury)
   - CT head/temporal bones (high resolution)
   - Facial palsy assessed with NCS (ENoG D3-21) and if >90% degeneration consider surgery
5. Management:
   - Conservative:
     - Eye care if CN VII injury
     - Hearing aids: BTE, bone conduction devices, MEI
     - Bed rest, head up 30°, laxatives etc. if CSF leak
   - Medical:
     - Steroid therapy for 1–2/52 if delayed CN VII palsy
     - Antibiotics for CSF leaks controversial. Advise pneumococcus, haemophilus and meningococcus vaccination
     - Vertigo: Vestibular suppressants <48 hrs (avoid long term as prevents compensation), physio
   - Surgical:
     - Hearing loss:
       - Exploration at 2 months if suspected ossicular discontinuity
     - Facial nerve paralysis: Immediate vs delayed onset
       - Await improvement, and if none, consider decompression at 2–3/52
       - Decompression if bony spicule identified as cause and immediate complete paralysis
       - If complete paralysis, and ENoG shows >90% between 3 and 21 days, explore
       - Approaches:

    - o Transmastoid/supralabyrinthine: If well aerated mastoid, requires OC dislocation (incus, which may already have taken place). Ideal in otic capsule sparing fractures. Avoids CNS exposure
    - o Translabyrinthine: Most common in otic capsule disrupting fractures, sacrifices hearing
    - o Middle fossa: If contra-lateral hearing loss, or normal hearing ipsilateral side
  - – Cholesteatoma post-trauma
    - • Implantation of skin into ME or ingrowth of entrapped epithelium at fracture site
  - – Vascular injury: ICA/IJV
    - • ICA: Pack ear, urgent angiogram, repair with stent or occlude?? Ligation in extremis

6. Evidence:
   - – Cochrane Database Systematic Review (2015): Antibiotic prophylaxis for preventing meningitis in patients with basilar skull fractures:
     - • No evidence for use of prophylactic antibiotics

Petrous Apex Lesions

1. Background:
   - – Usually benign smooth masses can be locally destructive due to expansile and compressive nature
2. History:
   - – Can be asymptomatic or nonspecific
   - – Signs of petrous apicitis
     - • Severe headache
     - • Ear: Otalgia hearing loss
     - • Eye: Retro-orbital pain, double vision
     - • CN6 palsy: Gradenigo's syndrome
     - • Facial palsy
3. Examination:
   - – Large lesions or those close to CN (e.g. Meckel cave, cavernous sinus, IAC) may cause CN palsies
     - • Commonly CN V/VI as susceptible to compression: Only thin layer of dura between CN and petrous apex
4. Investigations:
   - – MRI + Gd and fat saturation techniques
   - – CT scan: For asymmetric pneumatisation, and for some bony pathologies
   - – Diffusion-weighted imaging to distinguish cholesteatoma vs other diagnosis
   - – NB: Asymmetric pneumatisation is often mistaken for lesion on MRI

5. Management:
   - Conservative (watchful waiting) vs surgical
   - No hearing preservation
     - Translabyrinthine
   - Hearing preservation
     - Transpetrous
       - Infracochlear approach
       - Infralabyrinthine approach
     - MCF
     - Trans-sphenoidal
       - Increasing popularity can even be utilised when cyst is not abutting the sphenoid.

Causes and imaging characteristics of petrous apex lesions:

Lesions	*Imaging Characteristics*
Benign lesions	
Meningioma	Dural tail
Epidermoid cyst	Reduced intensity T1, increased T2 and DWI
Paraganglioma	Salt-and-pepper on MRI, permeation of bone
Mucocele	Opacification of petrous air cells and expansion of cortical margins on CT; hyperintense T2, variable T1
Langerhans cell histiocytosis	Destructive lesion
Arachnoid cyst (close to but not in petrous apex or in bone)	Reduced intensity T1, increased T2 and DWI
Malignant tumours	
Chondrosarcoma	Increased intensity T2 (most common solid lesion)
Chordoma	Honeycomb enhancement (usually midline)
Metastasis	

Developmental lesions	
Cholesterol granuloma	Increased intensity on T1 and T2, without fat saturation
Cephalocele	CSF signal intensity on all sequences
Congenital cholesteatoma	Restricted diffusion DWI
Inflammatory lesions	
Petrous apicitis	
Osteomyelitis	
Granulomatosis with polyangiitis	
Vascular lesions	
Petrous carotid aneurysm	
Intraosseous dural arteriovenous fistula	Multiple intraosseous flow voids

Chapter 4

Rhinology and Facial Plastics

Adnan Darr, Karan Jolly, Shahzada Ahmed and Claire Hopkins

Contents

DOI: 10.1201/9781003247098-4

Autoimmune Conditions in ENT

Granulomatosis with polyangiitis (GPA/Wegener's):	Eosinophilic granulomatosis with polyangiitis (Churg-Strauss):

• Small vessel necrotising vasculitis
• Involvement of upper (subglottis) and lower airway (90% respiratory)
• Septal perforation/saddling, crusting, ulceration, sinusitis
• Investigations:
  • Biopsy of affected organ during active disease (septal)
  • Pulmonary biopsy has the highest yield (VATS or open) > renal > septum
  • cANCA = Cytoplasmic anti-neutrophil cytoplasmic antibodies (PR3 = Proteinase-3), FBC, ESR, U&Es, LFTs
• Treatment:
  • Immunnosuppressants or monoclonal antibodies (eg rituximab)
  • Co-trimoxazole in patients due to colonisation with staph aureus
  • Surgical correction of nasal deformity only after 12 months of remission
	• Small vessel necrotising vasculitis
	• Triad of eosinophilia (>10% of total WCC), granuloma and vasculitis
	• Rhinosinusitis, septal lesions, polyps, hearing loss
	• Pulmonary involvement, mononeuritis, polyneuropathy
	• Cardiac complications: Myocarditis (50% of deaths from cardiac complication)
	• Investigations:
	  • eosinophilia, biopsy of affected organ or tissue
	  • p-ANCA to MPO (myeloperoxidase)
	  • CT sinuses and chest (pulmonary infiltrates)
	• Treatment with steroids and immunosuppressants or monoclonal antibodies (eg mepolizumab, benralizmab) in severe disease only

Sarcoidosis:
• Unknown aetiology, with granulomas (non-caseating)
• Mainly Caribbean females affected
• Multi-system disease
• Pulmonary involvement (88%)
• Lupus pernio
• Bilateral hilar lymphadenopathy
• Submucosal supraglottic lesions (epiglottis)
• Heerfordt's disease (fever, parotid swelling, CN VII palsy)
• Investigations:
  • Raised serum ACE and Ca levels
  • Biopsy of affected organ for diagnosis: Septal, lymph node or lung biopsy
  • CXR (BHL), CT chest
• Treatment:
  • Systemic steroids
	Rheumatoid arthritis:
	• Idiopathic autoimmune disease
	• Affects synovial joints (CAJ)
	• TMJ involvement, CAJ fixation, ossicular fixation
	• Subcutaneous nodules
	• Investigations:
	  • ANA, RF, anti-CCP, U&Es, LFTs
	  • Laryngeal EMG to distinguish between fixation and palsy
	• Treatment:
	  • Steroids, MTX, hydroxychloroquine, monoclonal antibodies (rituximab)

Systemic lupus erythromatosus (SLE):
• Autoimmune connective tissue disease
• Immune complex deposition in end organs
• Septal ulceration, oral lesions, lymphadenopathy, CAJ fixation, parotid enlargement
• Investigations:
  • ANA, anti-DsDNA, U&Es, LFTs
  • Biopsy is diagnostic
• Treatment:
  • Steroids
  • Hydroxychloroquine methotrexate, azathioprine
	Relapsing polychondritis:
	• Autoimmune disease affecting cartilaginous tissue
	• Deposition of glycosaminoglycans
	• Chondritis:
	  • Auricular, sparing lobule
	  • Respiratory (trachea)
	  • Nasal (saddle deformity)
	  • Polyarthritis
	  • Cardiac (valvular) involvement
	• Investigations:
	  • Raised ESR, IgG (type II and IV collagen)
	• Treatment:
	  • NSAIDs, steroids, dapsone

Sjogren's syndrome: • Systemic autoimmune condition • Deposition of lymphocytes within exocrine glands	

• Primary or secondary (associated with other autoimmune conditions i.e. RA)
• Association with NH-lymphoma
• Xerostomia, sialomegaly, keratoconjunctivitis sicca
• Investigations:
  • Schirmer's test: Norm = >15 mm/5 min
  • ANA, ESR, anti-Ro, ant-La
  • Lip/salivary gland biopsy is diagnostic
• Treatment:
  • Steroids
  • Immunosuppression
  • Monoclonal antibodies
  • IV Ig	

Facial Pain

1. Background:
2. History:
   - SOCRATES: S(ite), O(nset), C(haracter), R(adiation), A(ssociation), T(iming), E(xacerbating), S(everity)
   - Autonomic symptoms or neurological deficits
   - Nasal symptoms: Congestion, discharge, sinus barotrauma – timing of onset and fluctuations in severity relative to pain important
   - TMJ symptoms (clicking)
   - DH: Previous nasal steroid therapy or antibiotics
   - PMH: Depression, stress, bruxism
3. Examination: Usually negative unless sinonasal cause
   - FNE to rule out sinonasal pathology
   - Cranial nerve examination, particularly CNV
4. Management: See Table 4.1
5. Investigations:
   - XR/MRI in TMJ dysfunction
   - CT if sinonasal pathology suspected, ideally when patient is symptomatic if RAR suspected
   - MRI head if suspicion of trigeminal neuralgia, to rule out extrinsic compression (vascular loops)

Table 4.1 Facial Pain Pathology and Characteristic Features

Pathology	*Features*
Tension-type headache	• Bi-frontal or bi-temporal symptoms • Episodic (<15 days/month) or chronic (>15 days/month) • Dull and described as a tight band-like pain • Can be occipital due to muscular trigger points • Precipitated by stress • Treated with simple OTC analgesia or amitriptyline (10 mg nocte, up to 50 mg)
Midfacial segment pain	• Similar description to TTH, but retro-orbital, nasion or maxillary distribution • May have hyperaesthesia • Misdiagnosed as sinusitis • Treatment again with low dose Amitriptyline
Migraine	• Predominantly unilateral • 4–72 hrs • Preceding aura • May develop temporary neurological deficits and autonomic symptoms (epiphora, rhinorrhoea) • Treatment with simple analgesics or 5-HT1 agonists • Prophylaxis with pizotifen (0.5–1.5 mg OD) or propranolol (80–240 mg daily in divided doses)
TMJ dysfunction	• Localised to TMJ with bi-temporal radiation or radiation to neck • Associated with bruxism • Exacerbated by chewing, with focal area of pain • Degenerative joint disease or chronic myofascial pain (latter most common) • Treated with simple analgesics, steroids, stretch exercises
Trigeminal neuralgia	• Severe sharp radiating pain (V2 or V3) • Exacerbated when tapping over nerve distribution • Can be idiopathic or secondary to compression by vasculature or neoplasms o trigeminal ganglion, hence need for MRI scan • Carbamazepine is first-line medical treatment • Surgical treatment is decompression or gamma knife surgery

(Continued)

Table 4.1 Facial Pain Pathology and Characteristic Features ***(Continued)***

Pathology	*Features*
Trigeminal autonomic cephalgias	Group of conditions causing pain over the ophthalmic distribution of CN V, with autonomic symptoms (epiphora, rhinorrhoea and Horner syndrome)
1) Cluster headache	• Excruciating unilateral pain in retro or peri-orbital region • Short history (1 hr) • Male predominance • Treatment with oxygen initially and SC sumatriptan (6 mg), verapamil long-term
2) Paroxysmal hemicrania	• As above • Lasting up to 30 min • Female predominance • Up to 40 episodes per day • Treatment with indomethacin (25–75 mg TDS)
3) SUNCT (short unilateral neuralgiform headache with conjunctival injection and tearing) or SUNA (autonomic symptoms)	• Short lasting • Up to 200 attacks per day • Treatment with lamotrigine 100 mg OD or SC lidocaine
Atypical facial pain	• Diagnosis of exclusion • Associated with psychological distress

Septal Perforation

1. Background:
   - Causes:
     - Idiopathic
     - Iatrogenic (digital trauma, nasal cautery or surgery)
     - Infective (syphilis)
     - Autoimmune (GPA, sarcoidosis, SLE)
     - Medication (cocaine, decongestants, steroids)
     - Malignancy (SCC, midline T-cell lymphoma)
2. History:
   - History of presenting complaint:
     - Often asymptomatic
     - Congestion
     - Whistling

        - Crusting
        - Epistaxis
        - External deformity
    - Past medical history:
        - Nasal trauma
        - Previous nasal surgery (cautery, septoplasty/septorhinoplasty)
        - Systemic disorders
    - Drug history:
        - Substance misuse (cocaine)
        - Topical decongestant/steroid use
3. Examination:
    - Nasal flow: Whistling due to turbulent flow
    - Anterior rhinoscopy and flexible nasendoscopy to rule out malignancy. May demonstrate crusting/irregular edges, ulceration
    - Saddling/tip support compromise
4. Investigations:
    - Biopsy if suspected malignancy or diagnosis of GPA vasculitis (during active disease as yield low)
    - Urinalysis: Cocaine
    - Haematological:
        - FBC, U&Es (vasculitis), ESR, CRP, WCC
        - Ca, ACE (sarcoidosis)
        - cANCA for GPA (raised in acute phase) with PR3 (MPO with pANCA). May be weakly positive in cocaine use due to preservative Levamisole
        - Treponemal antibodies (syphilis)
        - RF and DsDNA (SLE)
    - CXR to assess for bilateral hilar lymphadenopathy
    - CT thorax may be warranted to assess for lung involvement in granulomatosis with polyangiitis
    - CT sinuses to assess for sinusitis extent and bony erosion
5. Management:
    - MDT approach usually involving respiratory, renal and rheumatological physicians if systemic cause
    - Conservative:
        - Observation if asymptomatic and incidental finding
    - Medical:
        - Saline irrigation
        - 25% glucose in glycerol drops for crusting
        - Barrier creams, petroleum-based ointments and nasal douching for crusting and dryness
    - Surgical:
        - Customised/non-customised septal obturator (customised requires CT scan)

- Small to medium perforations are only ones where surgical closure should be attempted – open/closed approach, although this is broadly based on level of experience
  - Free grafts (conchal cartilage): Failure high (50%) if >2 cm
  - Pedicled flap (nasoseptal, inferior turbinate)
  - Rotation/advancement using septal mucosa bilaterally
  - Interposition material (fascia, cartilage advancement, PDS plate)

Peri-orbital Cellulitis

1. Background:
   - Organism: Strep pneumoniae > haemophilus influenzae B > moraxella catarrhalis
   - Extension directly through thin lamina, through valveless venous system, lymphatics, congenital dehiscence
   - Orbital septum: Fibrous layer separating globe and skin, acting as infection barrier:
     - Superiorly from periosteum of orbital rim
     - Inferiorly to tarsal plate
2. History:
   - Duration of symptoms
   - Recent coryzal illness/URTI, sinusitis
   - Trauma (insect bite)
   - Eye symptoms: Pain, reduced acuity
   - Evidence of intracranial involvement: Meningism or reduced conscious level
3. Examination:
   - Ophthalmology:
     - Unilateral or bilateral eye symptoms
     - Extent of lid swelling, and whether eye opening is compromised
     - Chemosis/proptosis
     - Ophthalmoplegia/pain on eye movements. Afferent pupil defect (cranial nerve III). Colour vision/acuity (cranial nerve II) – Ishihara/Snellen chart (Kollner's rule: Red/green defects)
   - ENT:
     - Anterior rhinoscopy and FNE to assess middle meatus if permitted – polyps/purulent discharge, MC&S if possible
   - Neurology:
     - GCS, cranial nerve examination and Brudzinski/Kernig's test
   - Paediatric:
     - Seek paediatric review in children
4. Investigations:
   - Intravenous access, U&E's (for contrast), CRP, FBC, clotting profile
   - Middle meatal pus swab

  - CT scan, with contrast of paranasal sinuses and orbits ± head – triplanar views
  - MRI if CNS involvement (cerebritis), cavernous sinus thrombosis (CST) or palsies
5. Management:
  - MDT: Ophthalmology, paediatrics, neurosurgery ± neurosurgery if intra-cranial complications
  - Medical: This may be considered in the instances of a small subperiosteal abscess (<4 mm) and where regular close observation and immediate surgical intervention are available in the event of acute deterioration
    - Intravenous antibiotics as per local guidance (co-amoxiclav)
    - Topical nasal decongestants/steroid therapy
  - Surgical: In event of subperiosteal abscess:
    - Open approach (modified Lynch-Howarth/seagull) + limited ESS:
      - ■ Curvilinear incision below medial aspect of brow, down to periosteum/bone of medial orbit, until pus is encountered, with washout
      - ■ Pus for swabs for MC&S and corrugated drain inserted
      - ■ Endoscopic sinus surgery in acute setting is dependent on surgeon skill
  - Endoscopic approach:
    - Technically challenging due to acute inflammation
    - Reserved predominantly for adults due to anatomical consideration in paediatric population
    - Nasal decongestion
    - Uncinectomy, MMA, ethmoidectomy, breach of lamina and drainage of pus
    - Consider sphenoidotomy in presence of cavernous sinus thrombosis
6. Differential diagnoses:
  - Inflammatory: Bacterial/viral conjunctivitis, dacryocystitis
  - Skin: Contact dermatitis, HSV
  - Neoplasia: Rhabdomyosarcoma (particularly in paediatric population)

Chandler classification:

I	Pre-septal:	Lid oedema, erythema, chemosis
II	Post-septal:	Proptosis, chemosis, restricted gaze, afferent pupillary defect
III	Subperiosteal abscess:	Medial rectus oedema, displacement, antero-inferior globe displacement
VI	Orbital abscess:	Proptosis, chemosis, restricted gaze, no light perception
V	Cavernous sinus thrombosis:	Bilateral eye signs, headaches, swinging pyrexia

Note: Ophthalmoplegia from stage II and above

Cavernous sinus thrombosis:

- Cranial nerve involvement: 3, 4, V1, V2, 6
- Exophthalmos
- Bilateral eye swelling
- CNS irritation
- Papilloedema

Indications for CT:

- No improvement following min 24 hrs intravenous antibiotics
- Incomplete eye opening/unable to assess acuity/colour vision
- Bilateral eye symptoms ± swinging pyrexia (CST)
- Features of meningitis/intra-cranial spread (reduced GCS)
- Ophthalmoplegia (reduced acuity, colour vision loss, double vision, pain on gaze, restricted gaze)

Evidence:

- Oxford (O) et al. Medical and surgical management of subperiosteal orbital abscess secondary to acute sinusitis in children. Int J Pediatr Otorhinolaryngol. 2006; 70(11): 1853–1861 and Gavriel (G) et al. Dimension of subperiosteal orbital abscess as an indication for surgical management in children. Otolaryngol Head Neck Surg. 2011; 145(5): 823–827
  - Paediatric population
  - Most medial wall abscesses can be managed medically as long as:
    - No significant ophthalmoplegia, IOP < 20 mmHg, proptosis < 5 mm
  - Surgical management indicated if:
    - >17 mm length (G), >4 mm in width (G, O), Volume >0.5 mL (G)

Complications of Sinusitis: Pott's Puffy Tumour

1. Background:
   - Non-neoplastic complication of acute or chronic sinusitis/trauma
   - Common in adolescence
   - Acute sinusitis + anterior table erosion/osteomyelitis (± posterior table) + subperiosteal abscess
   - Secondary to frontal outflow obstruction (inflammatory/iatrogenic from previous surgery)
   - Strep viridans is the most common organism in complicated sinusitis

- Intra-cranial complications seen in 30% of cases
- Extension:
  - Directly (osteomyelitis)
  - Congenital dehiscence
  - Haematogenous (valveless veins)
  - Foramen of Breschet (drainage canals from frontal sinus)

2. History:
   - Duration of symptoms
   - Recent URTI
   - Nasal discharge/congestion
   - Previous history of ARS/CRS ± surgery
   - Systemic compromise
   - Headaches
3. Examination:
   - Anterior rhinoscopy/flexible nasendoscopy: Assessment of nasal polyps or obvious discharge emanating from frontal recess
   - Neurological assessment:
     - Cranial nerve assessment
     - Meningism
4. Investigations:
   - Cross-sectional imaging indications:
     - Neurological features (reduced GCS/emesis/meningism)
     - Obvious frontal sinus swelling, consistent with collection
   - CT head, paranasal sinuses, orbits and brain with contrast: Bony changes of anterior or posterior table and frontal recess
   - MRI in assessment of subtle intracranial extension, for cerebritis or early dural enhancement
5. Management:
   - Multi-disciplinary input: Neurosurgery in event of intra-cranial complications and microbiology in the event of poor response to intravenous therapy
   - Conservative: Saline douching
   - Medical:
     - Topical therapy: Decongestants and steroids
     - Intravenous antibiotics according to trust anti-microbial guidelines (usually Ceftriaxone with BBB crossover for 6/52)
   - Surgical:
     - Needle aspiration of pus to decompress + for MC&S
     - Endoscopic: Frontal sinus surgery/balloon sinuplasty
     - Open:
       - Frown line incision and abscess drainage
       - Frontal sinus trephine
       - Bi-coronal approach with neurosurgery if intracranial extension: Osteoplastic flap

- o Bicoronal incision with periosteum raised
- o Bone window created
- o Removal of frontal sinus mucosa as well as posterior table
- o Cranialization of frontal sinus
- o Pericranial flap, fascia or fat to seal off drainage pathway

Frontal sinus trephine:

- ■ With or without ESS with recess opening. Extended hot Draf procedures are associated with re-stenosis and may be considered at a later date:
  - Stab incision 1cm from midline at level of medial brow
  - Guide introduced and sinusotomy with drill (2 mm cutting burr)
  - Guide wire introduced into sinusotomy
  - Mini trephine introduced over wire + fluorescein confirmation endoscopically

Draf procedures:

- ■ Draf 1: Uncinectomy and complete anterior ethmoidectomy not disturbing the recess
- ■ Draf 2a: Lamina to middle turbinate
- ■ Draf 2b: Lamina to septum (includes head of middle turbinate)
- ■ Draf 3: Lamina to lamina (inter-sinus septum, nasal septum, to the anterior table and first olfactory filament)

Epistaxis

1. Background:
   - Anterior bleeds most commonly (90%) arise from Little's area/Kiesselbach's plexus: Vascular network formed by five arteries, derived from internal (anterior and posterior ethmoidal) and external (SPA, greater palatine, superior labial) carotid artery circulation
   - Posterior bleeds are usually less common, but most likely to lead to intervention/admission
   - Woodruff's plexus: Venous plexus located on lateral nasal wall below the inferior turbinate
     - Plexus is thin walled beneath a thin mucosa
2. History:
   - Recent coryzal episodes
   - Trauma (digital/falls)
   - Laterality/frequency/length of bleed and location (posterior or anterior)
   - History of bleeding diathesis/bruising

   - Treatment with antiplatelet/anticoagulants
   - History of illicit drug use
   - Red flags: Nasal congestion, ophthalmoplegia
3. Investigations:
   - FBC, U&E's, LFT's, clotting screen, G&S
4. Examination: Systematic ABCDE approach
   - Key concerns are:
     - Airway: Examine for clots in oropharynx and suction
     - Circulation: BP and tachycardia to assess for shock. Intravenous access and haematological profile as above
   - Rhinoscopy with aid of co-phenylcaine (5% lidocaine + 0.5% phenylephrine) if anterior bleed ± FNE if no anterior bleeding points identified
5. Management:
   - Conservative:
     - First aid measures including pressure, head positioning (forward) and cold press
   - Medical:
     - Intravenous fluids in cases of hypovolaemic shock
     - Floseal: Bovine derived gelatin matrix + human derived thrombin matrix, used in cases of diffuse ooze with no evidence of single site. A good option for elderly patients
     - Nasopore: Synthetic biodegradable fragmenting foam
     - Tranexamic acid
     - Chemical cautery with silver nitrate
     - Reversal of anticoagulation if required with vitamin K
   - Packing:
     - Anterior packing with Merocel or Rapid Rhino or Posterior packing with Foley catheter ± BIPP (be aware of toxic shock syndrome if left for >24 hrs or high-risk patient (immunocompromised). Commence antibiotics
     - See "Surgical management of epistaxis" for further details

- Causes:
  - Congenital: von Willebrand's disease, haemophilia, HHT
  - Traumatic/Iatrogenic: Digital trauma/surgery
  - Neoplasia:
    - Benign: IP, JNA
    - Malignant: Sinonasal, nasopharyngeal, lymphoma, leukaemia, myeloma
  - Systemic: Alcoholic liver disease, renal failure, ITP, HHT
  - Medications: Oral anticoagulants, antiplatelets, cocaine use

- Grades of shock:
  Grade I = 0–15% = Mild tachycardia
  Grade II = 15–30% = Moderate tachycardia, increased CRT
  Grade III = 30–40% = Hypotension, tachycardia, low output
  Grade IV = >40% = Profound hypotension

Surgical Management of Epistaxis

1. Endoscopic sphenopalatine artery ligation:
   - Bilateral occasionally as 15% have cross supply
   - Decongestion as per ESS (1:1000 adrenaline topically) with local anaesthetic infiltration of uncinate, axilla and head of middle turbinate
   - Middle turbinate medialised
   - Vertical incision is made 1 cm anterior to posterior attachment of middle turbinate
   - Mucoperiosteal flap is elevated and crista ethmoidalis is identified. SPA is posterior to this landmark
     - Alternatively, an antrostomy can be made, and the posterior fontanelle removed using through cutting forceps to visualise the back wall of the maxillary sinus as a surgical landmark
     - An indentation of the IMAX may be seen to guide surgeon to SPF
     - Flap is then elevated off the lateral wall to identify crista ethmoidalis and SPA
   - Kerrison's forceps may be used to remove crista ethmoidalis to provide additional length of the SPA
   - Ligation modalities must include bipolar or monopolar cautery as liga clips may displace intra or post-operatively
   - Mucoperiosteal flap is raised to face of sphenoid to identify multiple branches
   - Failure rate 15%, due to multiple branches (2/3 of patients have 2 or more branches)
2. Internal maxillary artery ligation:
   - Method used in failed cases of endoscopic sphenopalatine artery ligation
   - Decongestion as per ESS
   - Wide MMA
   - Posterior wall of maxillary sinus is removed with a drill/kerrison rongeur
   - Posterior periosteum incised
   - Internal maxillary artery identified within pad of fat and ligated with clips

3. Anterior ethmoidal artery (AEA) ligation if suspected trauma:
   - Lignospan infiltration
   - Lynch-Howarth incision
   - Subperiosteal elevation with freer or cottle elevator
   - Identification of lacrimal sac
   - AEA is 24 mm posterior to anterior lacrimal crest (PEA is 12 mm posterior to the AEA, Optic nerve is 6 mm posterior to PEA)
   - Artery ligated with clips or bipolar
4. External carotid artery ligation:
   - Incision two finger breadths below angle of mandible, dividing platysma and raising bilateral flaps
   - Dissect anterior border of SCM and retract to demonstrate carotid sheath
   - Identify CCA and place sling, dissect superiorly to bifurcation, and ECA is superficial and medial
   - NB: STA and APA must be identified before tying off ECA with Silk ties. Do not divide
5. Embolisation:
   - Usually reserved for patients unfit for general anaesthetic or failed SPA/IMAX ligation
   - Coiling, gelfoam, poly-vinyl-alcohol of IMAX (minimum 2 mm diameter vessels)
   - Risks include:
     - CVA
     - Cranial nerve neuropathies (mainly visual loss)
     - Facial pain
     - Skin loss

Moffat's solution:

- 1 mL 1:1000 adrenaline
- 2 mL 5% cocaine
- 2 mL 8.4% sodium bicarbonate

Hereditary Haemorrhagic Telangiectasia (Osler-Weber-Rendu Disease)

1. Background:
   - Autosomal dominant, usually presenting in late teens
   - Defect in TGF-β signaling pathway, resulting in deficient contractile tissue in vascular walls (tunica media) and angiogenesis
     - ENG (80% of cases) or ACVRL1 mutation

- Telangiectasia and AVMs (large vessel malformations occur in large organs including brain, lungs and liver)
- MADH4 mutation may result in colonic polyps in some patients, later transforming into colorectal cancer
- Higher risk of DVT

2. History:
   - Epistaxis manifests early and is present in 90% of patients
   - Respiratory system involvement may result in haemoptysis
   - Liver involvement may lead to portal hypertension and cirrhosis, with subsequent encephalopathy
   - Neurological involvement may result in headaches, seizures or a CVA (~1% risk/year)
   - High output can lead to congestive cardiac failure (CCF) due to shunting of blood from major organs, resulting in paroxysmal dyspnoea and orthopnoea
   - Black stools may be present due to haemorrhage from varices in upper or lower GI tract
3. Examination:
   - Telangiectasia is usually through direct examination:
     - Anterior rhinoscopy
     - Nasendoscopy
     - Oropharyngeal examination
     - Skin (fingers, face and ears)
4. Investigations:
   - Genetic screening is available, although clinical findings are sufficient
   - Haematological/biochemistry: FBC, iron and clotting to rule out other causes
   - Radiological: CTPA. MRA (brain, abdomen)
   - Cardiovascular: Bubble echo
   - Liver: Doppler USS, LFTs
   - GI: OGD/capsule endoscopy
5. Management:
   - MDT:
     - Geneticist, haematologist
   - Epistaxis:
     - Conservative:
       - ■ First aid for epistaxis
       - ■ Nasal emollients
     - Medical:
       - ■ Blood transfusions/iron supplementation
       - ■ Emollients
       - ■ Tranexamic acid (oral)
       - ■ Oestrogenic creams
       - ■ Anti-VEGF: Avastin infusion (bevacizumab)

- Surgical:
  - ■ Nasal obturator
  - ■ Packing with non-traumatic methods such as Kaltostat or Nasopore
  - ■ Cautery (attempt to avoid)
  - ■ KTP laser or coblation
  - ■ Septodermoplasty/Saunders procedure (use of split thickness skin graft (STSG) over debrided epithelial layer)
  - ■ Young's procedure to reduce airflow over septal mucosa (remain sealed as for 6/12 for atrophic rhinitis, 12–26 months HHT):
    - o Circumferential incision 1 cm inside alar rim
    - o Elevated mucosa is sutured to close the nasal vestibule (modified with anterior and posterior flaps sutured)

Curacao criteria (3/4 high likelihood, 2/4 low likelihood):

- ■ Family history
- ■ Telangiectasia (multiple)
- ■ AVM (lung, liver, brain)
- ■ Epistaxis (recurrent and spontaneous)

Evidence:

- ■ Cochrane (2016): Effect of Topical Intranasal Therapy on Epistaxis Frequency in Patients with Hereditary Haemorrhagic Telangiectasia: A Randomized Clinical Trial
  - – Insufficient evidence to suggest benefit of topical TXA, Oestriol or Avastin

Obstructive Sleep Apnoea (Adults)

1. Background:
   - – Male > Female
   - – 20% of population have mild OSA if BMI 25–30
   - – Collapse of airway secondary to Bernoulli principle: Flow of air through a narrow aperture must increase in velocity, resulting in a pressure drop
   - – Terminology:
     - Apnoea: Cessation of flow for 10 secs with effort (pauses in breathing)
     - Hypopnea: 50% flow reduction for 10 secs or reduction of sats by 4% with effort (shallow breathing)
     - Obstructive sleep apnoea syndrome (OSAS) = OSA with symptoms
     - Upper airway resistance syndrome (UARS) = Features of OSA with normal AHI

- Increased risk of arrhythmias (sinus brady), CVA, IHD, hypertension, CCF (cor pulmonale), pulmonary artery hypertension, insulin resistance, GORD, intracranial hypertension

2. History:
   - Initial assessment with Epworth sleepiness scale (0–10 is normal):
   - History of presenting complaint:
     - Snoring
     - Witnessed apnoea
     - Weight gain, daytime somnolence
   - PMH: Weight, cardiovascular history, hypothyroidism, acromegaly
   - SH: Smoking, drinking
   - DH: Sedatives
3. Examination:
   - BMI
   - Mouth:
     - Mouth opening, overbite or underbite, retrognathia, macroglossia, tonsil size and Mallampati grading
   - Neck circumference: >17″ male and 15.5″ female most predictive indicator
   - Flexible nasendoscopy:
     - Mueller manoeuvre: Degree of retro-palatal and retro-lingual collapse on inspiration with nose and mouth closed, awake and supine (>50% abnormal)
     - Assess for polyps, septal deflection and adenoidal hypertrophy
4. Investigations:
   - Polysomnography: Video footage of EEG, electrooculography (stages of sleeping), nasal/oral flow, chest/abdominal expansion, HR, sats, CO_2 and EMG (for parasomnias). Will not show level of obstruction
   - Domiciliary sleep study: Portable device. Will not measure EEG, EOG, EMG or CO_2
5. Management:
   - Conservative/lifestyle: Reduction in alcohol, weight loss, smoking cessation, discontinue sedatives, positional modification, mandibular advancement device
   - Medical: CPAP (reduces morbidity and mortality)
   - Surgery: Will improve, but not cure symptoms – lack of high-quality evidence
     - Nasopharyngeal: Adenoidectomy, maxillary advancement (nasopharyngeal stenosis or collapse). Septoplasty will increase compliance and reduce pressure requirements
   - Oro/velopharyngeal: Tonsillectomy (treatment of choice in paediatric patients) ± UPPP, palatal stiffening procedures (implants, RF ablation, sclerosant), lateral pharyngoplasty

- Hypopharyngeal: Tongue base reduction/lingual tonsillectomy (coblation, RF, cautery, TORS), midline glossectomy, genioglossal advancement, hyoid suspension (releasing infra-hyoid muscles and re-attaching to mandible or thyroid cartilage)
- Mandibular/midface advancement
- NB: In event of excessive daytime somnolence, patients should be advised to stop driving and notify DVLA. Backed with clinical assessment (ESS and sleep studies)

Apnoea hypopnea index:

AHI = (Apnoea + Hypopnea)/h of sleep

Normal	0–5
Mild:	5–15
Moderate:	15–30
Severe:	>30

Epworth sleepiness scale:

- Eight questions, with score of 0–3, with max score of 24
- Likelihood of falling asleep during routine activities, 0 – none, 1 – slight, 2 – moderate, 3 – high

0–10:	Normal
11–15:	Mild to moderate OSA
16+:	Severe OSA

Olfactory Dysfunction

1. Background:
   - Anosmia: Absence of smell
   - Can be conductive or sensorineural
   - Hyposmia: Reduced sense of smell
   - Phantosmia: Phantom smells in the absence of a source/stimulus
   - Age related loss of smell is termed presbyosmia
   - Parosmia: distortion of smell in response to stimulus
2. History:
   - Duration of symptoms (age of onset would indicate a congenital or acquired pathology)
   - Taste disturbances (most flavour perception derived from smell; ask about true taste eg sweet, salty, sour tastes)
   - Recent URTI
   - Nasal congestion, discharge/rhinorrhea
   - History of trauma/falls

- PMH: Previous sinonasal surgery (see table of differentials)
- Medications and illicit drug use
- SH: Smoking
- Occupation: Chef?
- Household protection? Smoke alarms

3. Examination:
   - Cranial nerve assessment (neurological pathology)
   - Anterior rhinoscopy and flexible nasendoscopy:
     - Nasal polyposis
     - Rhinitis
     - Neoplasia
4. Investigations:
   - Haematological: U&Es (autoimmune involvement), LFTs, TFTs (hypothyroidism as cause), B12, folate, autoimmune screen
   - CT in the presence of polyps if ESS being considered
   - MRI to assess anterior cranial fossa:
     - Congenital loss
     - Idiopathic nature
     - Phantosmia (epilepsy protocol)
   - Olfactory testing UPSIT, sniffin sticks, odour threshold testing
5. Management:
   - Largely conservative:
     - Smell retraining kits
     - Support groups
     - Household advice:
       - Food expiration dates
       - Smoke alarms
   - Medical:
     - Topical in cases of proven CRS
     - Oral steroid trial in post-viral cases (lack of high-level evidence) after risk vs benefits have been discussed

- Causes:
  - Idiopathic
  - Iatrogenic: Surgery (ESS) or radiotherapy
  - Trauma: Skull base
  - Inflammatory: Chronic rhinosinusitis
  - Infection: Viral URTI (including COVID-19)
  - Systemic: GPA, sarcoidosis, thyroid disease, diabetes mellitus
  - Neurological: Parkinson's disease, multiple sclerosis, Alzheimer's disease
  - Congenital: Kallman's syndrome (lifelong hyposmia)

- Medications: Methotrexate, carbimazole, metronidazole, chemotherapy, cocaine
- Neoplastic:
  - Benign: Juvenile angiofibroma, meningioma, pituitary adenoma
  - Neoplastic: Nasopharyngeal Ca, sinonasal Ca, esthesioneuroblastoma

UPSIT:

- Four booklets, each consisting of ten odorants
- Specific to American odours, but used internationally
- Scratch and sniff, with four options per book – patient must answer even if they cannot recognise/identify smell
- Maximum score of 40
- Score relative to age and sex of matched controls
- Normosmia, hyposmia, anosmia or malingering
- Random/chance scoring will give 10/40, thus a score <5 suggests malingering. Hyposmia is defined between 5 and 15

Chronic Rhinosinusitis

1. Background
   - Characterised as with or without polyps
   - Inflammation of nose/sinus with two or more symptoms:
     - One must be:
       - Nasal congestion
       - Rhinorrhea/PND
     - ±reduced sense of smell OR facial pains
   - AND either:
     - Endoscopic signs of polyps, middle meatal oedema or middle meatal mucopus
   - AND/OR
     - CT evidence of sinus disease
   - Symptoms persist for >12 weeks
2. History
   - Symptoms of CRS (as above)
   - Duration, progression and laterality of symptoms
   - Allergic history (itchy/watery eyes/nose)
   - Nasal surgery or medication
   - PMH: Asthma, aspirin sensitivity, cystic fibrosis, PCD
3. Examination:
   - Rhinoscopy and FNE/rigid endoscopy

4. Investigations:
   - CT sinus: If no improvement on appropriate medical therapy:
     - Surgical planning and anatomy
     - Extent of disease
5. Management:
   - Conservative:
     - Nasal douching
   - Medical:
     - First-line topical steroids (drops/sprays)
     - Antihistamine if allergic features
     - eg polypoid middle turbinate
     - Oral steroid course in severe symptomatic cases (no more than 2/3 per year)
     - Antibiotics:
       - Non type 2: Eosinophils/IgE normal = macrolides
       - Type 2: Eosinophils/IgE elevated = EPOS 20 not recommended
   - Surgery
     - ESS ± polypectomy
       - Reduce inflammatory load
       - Better topical access
       - Symptom control

Paediatric population:

- CRS classification: Cough replaces smell
- With polyps think Cystic Fibrosis

Meltzer grading polyps:

- Grade 1: Confined to middle meatus (MM)
- Grade 2: Occupying MM up to MT
- Grade 3: Past MT
- Grade 4: Obstructing nasal cavity

Surgical risks

- Bleeding, infection, septal perforation (if combined with septoplasty), anosmia, orbital injury, visual loss, CSF leak, recurrence and further surgery

Nasal Polyposis

1. Background:
   - Inflammatory polyps: Type 2 inflammation (IL4, IL5, IL13 = Eosinophils and IgE
     - CRS
     - Aspirin exacerbated respiratory disease (AERD)

    - Allergic fungal rhinosinusitis (AFRS)
  - Cystic fibrosis
  - PCD
  - Eosinophilic GPA (triad of asthma, eosinophilia, rhinosinusitis)
2. History:
   - Nasal congestion, rhinorrhea, anosmia, facial pain
   - Duration, progression, laterality and severity of symptoms
   - Allergic history
   - Samters triad for AERD: Aspirin sensitivity, polyps, asthma
   - Red flags: Bleeding, facial numbness, visual symptoms
3. Examination:
   - FNE/Rigid endoscopy
   - Head and neck examination in suspected unilateral polyposis
4. Investigations:
   - RAST or skin prick if allergy suspected
   - CT sinuses
   - ANCA/ESR if suspecting vasculitis (EGPA)
   - Sweat test for CF
   - Saccharin test/mucosal biopsy for PCD (normal ciliary frequency 10–20 per second)
5. Management:
   - Conservative: Saline rinse
   - Medical:
     - Topical nasal steroids
     - Consider oral steroids (no more than 2× yearly)
       - 0.5 mg/kg prednisolone for 1 week
     - Antibiotics: Limited evidence for doxycycline
     - Aspirin desensitisation post surgery in AERD
   - MABs (currently licensed in USA and Europe only)
   - Surgery:
     - ESS
     - Will need post-operative medical management

AERD:

- Abnormal arachidonic acid metabolism pathway
- Excess leukotrienes
- Asthma, polyps, aspirin sensitivity
- Low salicylate diet
- Aspirin desensitisation post-operatively, within hospital setting
  - Build up dose of aspirin until no reaction
  - Maintenance on high doses i.e. 300–500 mg
  - Reduced recurrence/better symptom control, asthma control

Allergic Rhinitis

1. Background:
   - Sensitisation: Antigen presenting cells to helper T2 cells (CD4) → IL4+IL13
     - B-cell differentiation to plasma cells → IgE
   - Primary phase: Type 1 hypersensitivity reaction
     - 5–15 min
     - Mast cell degranulation = Histamine and prostaglandin/leukotrienes
   - Secondary phase:
     - After 4 hrs
     - Cytokine and IL5 promotes inflammation = Eosinophils and neutrophils
2. History:
   - Nasal symptoms
   - Atopy (itching, sneezing, epiphora)
   - Seasonal vs perennial and exacerbating factors
   - PMH: Asthma, atopy
   - Allergies: Seasonal allergies
   - Social history: Occupation, pets and smoking
3. Examination:
   - Rhinoscopy: IT hypertrophy, oedema of MT
   - Nasal airflow
   - Flexible or rigid endoscopy: Congestion, polyps, mucopus
   - Atopic features
4. Investigations:
   - Total IgE, RAST
   - Skin prick test:
     - Assesses sensitisation not allergy
     - Lancet used to prick skin through allergen suspension
     - Measure wheal after 10–15 min
       - Positive control: Histamine
       - Negative control: Preservative/saline
     - >3 mm negative control is positive
5. Management:
   - Conservative:
     - Allergen avoidance
     - Nasal douching
   - Medical: Stepwise approach: Depends whether intermittent/persistent – look at BSACI guidance
     - First line: Oral antihistamine
     - Second line: Intranasal steroids
     - Combined topical steroid + antihistamine (Dymista)
     - PO steroids (rarely) for crisis i.e. exams/performance

- Alternative treatments:
  - If asthmatic, then leukotriene receptor antagonist i.e. montelukast 10 mg OD
  - Mast cell stabilisers i.e. topical sodium cromoglycate drops
- Immunotherapy:
  - Licensed for tree/grass pollen and house dust mite allergies
  - Subcutaneous therapy:
    - Anaphylaxis risk: Hospital attendance
    - Weekly injection for 3 months then monthly for 3 yrs
  - Sublingual therapy:
    - First dose within hospital setting
    - Daily drops for 3 yrs

– Surgery:
  - Inferior turbinate reduction: Cautery, laser, turbinectomy, turbinoplasty. Little high-level evidence to advocate one modality over other

ARIA classification:

- Intermittent = <4 days/week or 4 weeks/year
- Persistent = >4days/week or 4 weeks/year
- Mild = sleep, work, social activities not affected
- Mod/severe = sleep, work, social activities affected

Topical steroid absorption:

- Fluticasone = 0.5%
- Mometasone = 0.5%
- Budesonide = 33% (could be used in pregnancy)
- Beclomethasone = 44%
- Betamethasone = 100%

Fungal Sinusitis

1. Background:
   – Invasive (acute, chronic or granulomatous) vs non-invasive (mycetoma or allergic fungal rhinosinusitis)
   – In invasive, the key is length of symptoms: Acute (<4/52) vs chronic or granulomatous (3/12)
   – *Aspergillus* fungal hyphae branch at 45 degrees, Rhizopus and Mucor at 90 degrees
2. History:
   – Timing and onset of symptoms is key (rapid vs lengthy)
   – Symptoms of allergic rhinitis

  - Headaches and neurological symptoms (cranial neuropathies)
  - PMH: Immunocompromised state (chemotherapy, HIV, DM)
  - DH: Treatment with steroids without any alleviation in symptoms
3. Examination:
  - Rhinoscopy/FNE as per examination of patient with CRS
  - Addition of oral examination in immunocompetent patient
  - Neurological examination if suspected invasive fungal sinusitis (reduced GCS or CN palsies)
4. Investigations:
  - U&E's, LFT's, CRP, ESR, FBC, clotting profile as well as glucose and HbA1c (glycaemic control)
  - Swab for MC&S
  - CT sinuses ± head: Bony erosion or double density in AFRS (Mn, Ca, Fe presence in allergic mucin)
  - MRI if suspicion of orbital/intracranial involvement
5. Management: See Table 4.2

Table 4.2 Invasive vs Non-Invasive Sinusitis Overview

Invasive	*Non-Invasive*

Acute invasive fungal sinusitis (Mucormycosis):
• *Aspergillus, Saprophyticus* (*Mucor, Rhizopus, Absidia*)
• Immunocompromised patients (diabetes, HIV, chemotherapy)
• High mortality (50%), with CNS involvement
• History:
  • Rapid symptom onset of sinusitis
• Examination:
  • Necrotic areas (eschar): Middle and inferior turbinate and septum
  • Palatal ulceration
  • Reduced bleeding on contact
  • Reduced sensation
• CT and MRI (intra-cranial extension – high signal on T2)
• Treatment: MDT approach with medical team
  • ESS + debridement until normal tissue seen
  • IV Amphotericin B (Mucor) or Voriconazole (*Aspergillus*)
  • Diabetic control/immunity control
	Mycetoma:
	• ABC: *Aspergillus* (common), *Bipolaris* and *Curvularia*
	• Immunocompetent patients
	• May have facial hypoesthesia
	• Unilateral sinus disease on CT (mainly maxillary, with osteitis)
	• Large MMA required
	• No long-term F/U required

(Continued)

Table 4.2 Invasive vs Non-Invasive Sinusitis Overview *(Continued)*

Invasive	*Non-Invasive*

Chronic invasive fungal sinusitis:
• 12/52 history
• *Aspergillus fumigatus*
• DM or patients on steroids, elderly, mildly immunocompromised, HIV
• Less cases of CN involvement or invasion into orbit
• Treatment as with acute invasive
• Both require follow-up due to recurrence
	Allergic fungal rhinosinusitis:
	• Similar organisms as mycetoma
	• Unilateral and asymmetric involvement of sinuses
	• Symptoms of CRS resistant to medical treatment
	• Raised IgE and eosinophilia
	• Bent and Kuhn classification (2/5 required):
	  • Eosinophilic mucin (eosinophils, Charcot-Leyden crystals, necrotic material, fungal hyphae)
	  • Non-invasive hyphae
	  • Polyposis
	  • Radiographic findings
	  • Type-1 hypersensitivity
	• Double density on CT
	• Treatment: As per CRS
	  • ESS + oral and topical steroids
	  • Long-term follow-up due to recurrence
	  • Oral Itraconazole, but must monitor LFTs
	  • Amphotericin washouts

Granulomatous invasive fungal sinusitis: • 12/52 history • *Aspergillus flavus* • Endemic to Africa, Pakistan and India • Non-caseating granuloma, fibrosis and Langerhans cells seen • Present with rapidly increasing mass • Good prognosis with low likelihood of recurrence	

6. Evidence:
   - Cochrane (2018): Topical or systemic anti-fungal therapy for allergic rhinosinusitis (fungal)
     - Low quality evidence, no clear benefit suggested

Mixed density sign:

- Fungal sinusitis
- Inverted papilloma
- Chondrosarcoma
- Ossifying fibroma

Endoscopic Sinus Surgery and Radiology

- Paranasal sinus development attributed to lateral nasal wall ridges (ethmoturbinals)
  - First ethmoturbinal: Ascending portion agger nasi; Descending portion uncinate process
  - Second ethmoturbinal: Middle turbinate
  - Third ethmoturbinal: Superior turbinate
  - Fourth and fifth fuse; Supreme turbinate if present
- Ethmoid system can be divided into lamellae: In order of structure encountered when undertaking an ethmoidectomy
  - First: Uncinate process
  - Secon: Ethmoid bulla
  - Third: Basal lamella
  - Fourth: Superior turbinate
    - AEA is found between the second and third lamella, behind the face of the bulla unless a suprabulbar recess is present
- Messerklinger landmarks:
  - Four consistent:
    - Uncinate process
    - Ethmoid bulla anterior wall
    - Middle turbinate basal lamella
    - Face of sphenoid
  - Three inconsistent:
    - Ethmoid bulla posterior wall
    - Superior turbinate basal lamella
    - Supreme turbinate basal lamella
- ESS complications
  - Bleeding: 5%
  - Orbital injury: 1:500
  - CSF leak: 1:1500

- Interpreting CT images: CLOSET:
  C(ribriform plate) + C(arotid) – Keros classification
  L(amina) papyracea (dehiscence)
  O(ptic nerve) + O (nodi cell = sphenoethmoidal cell, postero-lateral, close to ICA and optic nerve)
  S(phenoid) sinus (pneumatisation, septation, attachment to cavernous carotid segment)
  E(thmoid) artery (Kennedy's nipple, low lying or along skull base)
  T(eeth) (Odontogenic sinusitis)
  Coronal plane: Septum, optic nerve, skull base, anterior ethmoidal artery, Onodi and Haller (infra-orbital cell)
  Sagittal plane: Frontal sinus and recess, skull base

Frontal recess landmarks:

Anterior:	Agger nasi (most anterior ethmoid air cell)
Medial:	Middle turbinate
Lateral:	Lamina
Posterior:	Face of ethmoid bulla

International Frontal Sinus Anatomy classifications (IFAC):

Cells	***Cell name***	***Definition***
Anterior cells (frontal sinus drainage pathway pushed posterior and medially).	Agger nasi cell	Cell that sits anterior to the insertion of the middle turbinate
	Supra agger cell	Anterior-lateral ethmoidal cell above ANC not pneumatizing into frontal sinus
	Supra agger frontal cell	Anterior-lateral ethmoidal cell pneumatizing into the frontal sinus
Posterior cells (frontal sinus drainage pathway pushed anteriorly)	Supra bulla cell	Cell above bulla ethmoidalis not entering the frontal sinus

(Continued)

Cells	*Cell name*	*Definition*
	Supra bulla frontal cell	Cell that pneumatizes from the suprabullar space into the frontal sinus
	Supraorbital ethmoid cell	An anterior ethmoid cell that pneumatizes around, anterior to or posterior to the AEA over the roof of the orbit
Medial cells (frontal sinus drainage pathway pushed lateral)		Medially based cell of the anterior ethmoid or the inferior frontal cell attached to or located in the interfrontal sinus septum

Keros classification of olfactory depth:

I: 1–3 mm
II: 4–7 mm
III: 8 mm+
IV: Asymmetric skull base

- Risk of skull base injury is higher with ascending grade
- Lateral lamella is the most common site of an iatrogenic CSF leak

Sphenoid sinus pneumatisation:

Conchal
Pre-sellar
Sellar
Post-sellar

Lund McKay scoring system on CT: Total score of 24

- Middle meatus, maxillary, frontal, anterior and posterior and sphenoid sinuses (right and left = 12)
- Score: 0 = no disease, 1 = Partial disease, 2 = Complete opacification (NB middle meatus is 0 or 2)

Complications of Endoscopic Sinus Surgery: Retrobulbar Haemorrhage

1. Background:
   - Usually due to retraction after avulsion of AEA
   - Can also be due to venous bleed from injury near lamina papyracea

- Raised intra-orbital pressure compresses vascular supply to optic nerve
- Permanent blindness can occur within 60–90 min if untreated
- Prevention:
  - Ensure eyes are not covered intra-operatively
  - Pre-operative evaluation of CT:
    - Supraorbital cell, resulting in AEA lying within mesentery below skull base
    - Oblique skull base
    - Bony dehiscence

2. Examination:
   - Ecchymosis
   - Proptosis
   - Conjunctival changes (chemosis)
   - RAPD
   - Palpable tenseness
   - If patient awake, then disproportionate pain
   - Tonometry: Intraocular pressures are very useful (normal IOP: 10–20 mmHg)
3. Management:
   - MDT: Ophthalmology
   - Conservative:
     - Orbital massage and ice application
   - Medical:
     - Intravenous dexamethasone 0.15–0.30 mg/kg
     - Mannitol 1 g/kg
     - Acetazolamide 500mg BD
     - Intravenous tranexamic acid
   - Surgical:
     - Control hemorrhage internally with bipolar if possible
     - Lateral canthotomy
       - Lidocaine subcutaneously at lateral canthus then hemostat to clamp lateral canthus
       - Incision through the skin at the lateral canthus down to the lateral orbital rim
       - Identify lateral canthal tendon and incise vertically, releasing inferior limb
       - Lower eyelid should be easily distracted from the globe and overlap partially over the upper eyelid
     - Medial external (Lynch)
     - Medial orbital wall decompression (endoscopic) should be considered especially in the event of inadequate response i.e. persistent tense globe/raised IO pressure
       - Linear incisions of periorbita (fat should prolapse into nasal cavity)

Complications of Endoscopic Sinus Surgery: Internal Carotid Artery Bleed

1. Background/Anatomy of ICA:
   - Starts at carotid bifurcation @ C4
   - Carotid sinus just superior to starting point
   - Posterior to ECA
   - Ascends on pharyngeal wall and pharyngobasilar fascia
   - Cincinnati classification: Seven segments, which can be subdivided according to location
   - Bleeds most common at the left paraclinoid segment
   - Lt > Rt
   - There is typically 1 l of blood loss per minute
   - Even when controlled, permanent neurological sequelae can persist
2. History:
   - Usually associated with previous radiotherapy patients and functioning pituitary adenomas with cavernous involvement
   - May have a history of previous surgery/incomplete resection of tumour, hence scar tissue and altered anatomy
3. Examination:
   - May be an ooze, or a profuse bleed obscuring vision within seconds
4. Management:
   - MDT approach: Anaesthetist, assistant surgeon, remaining theatre team, interventional radiologist all must be notified
   - Activate major haemorrhage protocol (criteria of >150 mL/h, >50%/3 hrs or circulating volume loss/24 hrs)
   - Consider conservative measures:
     - Suction × 2 to improve surgical field
     - Compression of ipsilateral neck
   - Medical:
     - Consider TXA and inform anaesthetic colleagues
   - Surgical:
     - Packing with ribbon gauze
     - Crushed muscle patch to be harvested by second surgeon: SCM, temporalis fascia, vastus lateralis from thigh, which contains thrombogenic properties. Placed over defect with gentle pressure for 10 min
     - If no improvement, pack and transfer to interventional radiology for angiogram:
       - ■ Options include:
         - o Balloon occlusion/embolization
         - o Coiling

- If poor collateral circulation, stent
  - Risks:
    - 20% risk of mortality
    - 50% risk of CVA
- ■ Post-operatively:
  - Repeat angiography at 24 and 72 hrs, and if no evidence of pseudoaneurysm or ongoing bleed, then packing removed and patient extubated
- ICA ligation in the neck is a last resort

Cincinnati classification:

C1: Cervical

Petrous segments:

C2: Petrous
C3: Lacerum

Cavernous segment:

C4: Cavernous

Intra-cranial segments:

C5: Clinoid
C6: Ophthalmic (supra-clinoid)
C7: Communicating

Major haemorrhage protocol:

- ■ 6421 ratio
  - Six units of RCC
  - Four units of FFP
  - Two units of cryoprecipitate
  - One unit of platelets

CSF Rhinorrhoea

1. Background:
   - Most common site for CSF leaks: Lateral cribriform plate lamella
   - Causes:
     - Spontaneous associated with IIH
     - Iatrogenic: ESS (1:1500)
     - Inflammatory: Acute invasive fungal sinusitis

  - Neoplastic: Invasive
  - Tegmen via eustachian tube
  - Idiopathic
2. History:
   - Duration of onset and site
   - Exacerbating factors: OSA, chronic cough
   - History of meningitis
   - PMH: Trauma or sinus surgery
3. Examination:
   - Flexible nasendoscopy: Site of leak may be difficult to localise, but may see a meningocele
   - Ear examination: Unilateral effusion in lateral skull base defect
   - Neurological examination: Cranial nerve palsy suggestive of raised ICP (cranial nerve 6)
   - Halo sign: Blood mixed with CSF on tissue. CSF will move by capillary action further peripherally than blood
4. Investigations:
   - High resolution CT scan skull base and temporal bones in initial instance to assess for bony defects in skull base (85%)
   - T2 weighted MRI for meningoencephalocele or fluid within sinuses. In combination with CT scan localise in 95% of cases
   - Myelogram (CT) with intrathecal gadolinium contrast evaluates sub-arachnoid space and may demonstrate an empty sella but is more invasive and less common
   - Radionuclide cisternography for low flow leaks: Indium-111 DTPA scintigraphy – injected via spinal tap, with images acquired at 6 and 24 hrs
   - β2-transferrin-assay (gold standard): 0.5–1 mL of nasal fluid required
     - Usually present exclusively in CSF
     - Can also be found in aqueous humour and perilymph
     - May be present in alcoholic liver disease
     - Serum sample must be taken as certain conditions may have raised serum β2 transferrin levels
   - Can also use β2-trace protein, found in choroid plexus, with CSF concentration 35× level in serum
5. Management:
   - MDT approach with neurosurgical team
   - Conservative:
     - Reserved for isolated post-traumatic cases, with short history of up to 10 days
     - Bed rest, with head at 45 degrees

    - Methods to reduce strain i.e. stool softeners, antitussives
  - Medical:
    - Pneumovax, Hib and meningococcal
  - Surgical: Gold standard endoscopic, endonasal:
    - Lumbar puncture and combination of 0.2–0.3 mL of 10% fluorescein (100 mg/mL) and 10 mL CSF, to be infused intrathecally to localise leak (unlicensed)
    - Depends on size of defect and location, but many different techniques exist:
      - ■ <1 cm and low flow leaks: Generally, overlay technique of free mucosal graft, fascial graft or fat plug
      - ■ >1 cm and high flow: Dural graft or fascial inlay with free mucosal overlay or vascularised pedicled flap (NSF)
    - 24 hrs intravenous antibiotics and bed rest followed by mobilisation
    - Consider measuring opening pressures post-operatively to identify patients with IIH for ongoing treatment (e.g. acetazolamide, VP shunting, ophthalmology review)
    - Follow-up in 6/52 and nasal saline irrigation after 1/52

6. Evidence:
   - Cochrane Database (2011): No evidence for prophylactic antibiotic use in prevention of meningitis

IIH:

- ■ F > M, with raised BMI
- ■ Chronically raised ICP, with raised CSF pressure (8–15 mmHg or 100–180 mmH_2O)
- ■ Papilloedema: 3C's (cupping, contour and colour)
- ■ Unilateral or bilateral cranial nerve 6 palsy should be only neurological sign
- ■ Empty sella (widening of the ST due to raised CSF pressure = pituitary compression/half-moon appearance)
- ■ Patulous optic nerve on MRI
- ■ MRV should be undertaken to rule out dural venous sinus thrombosis

Beta-2-Transferrin:

- ■ Aqueous humour
- ■ CSF
- ■ Perilymph

Mucocoele

1. Background:
   - Most common expansile mass within sinuses, resulting in bony resorption/erosion due to sinus outflow obstruction
   - Benign cystic masses encased by respiratory epithelium (pseudostratified ciliated columnar), with mucous accumulation
   - Frontal > ethmoid > maxillary > sphenoid
   - Fluctuating eye symptoms, think mucopyocoele
   - Causes:
     - Iatrogenic: Previous surgery or trauma
     - Inflammatory: Allergy, CRS or ARS
     - Neoplastic obstruction: Polyposis, JNA, osteoma, ossifying fibroma, fibrous dysplasia, sinonasal malignancy
     - Congenital: Craniofacial abnormalities i.e. craniosynostosis (Apert's, Crouzon's, Pfeiffer)
2. History:
   - HPC:
     - Nasal congestion/discharge/facial pain (rhinosinusitis)
     - Diplopia/visual compromise (extrinsic compression), which settle following surgery and bony re-modelling
     - Swelling over affected region, along with length of symptoms
     - Headaches (sphenoid mucocoele)
     - Systemic compromise: Pyocoele or meningitis (posterior table erosion as thinner than the anterior table)
   - PMH:
     - Trauma/sinus or neurosurgery surgery
3. Examination:
   - Head and neck examination: Swellings, proptosis and globe displacement (Figure 4.1)
   - Full cranial nerve examination: Focusing on visual acuity, eye movements, pain on restriction and reflexes
   - Anterior rhinoscopy:
     - Start with nasal flow, and assess for obvious polyp disease and discharge
   - Flexible nasendoscopy/rigid endoscopy with 3 pass technique following nasal decongestion to evaluate middle meatus and PNS
4. Investigations:
   - CT scan:
     - Will determine relationship with neighbouring structures and aid surgical planning
     - Shows non-rim enhancing lesion (unless pyocoele). Homogenous and isotense
     - Expansion and bony remodelling also seen

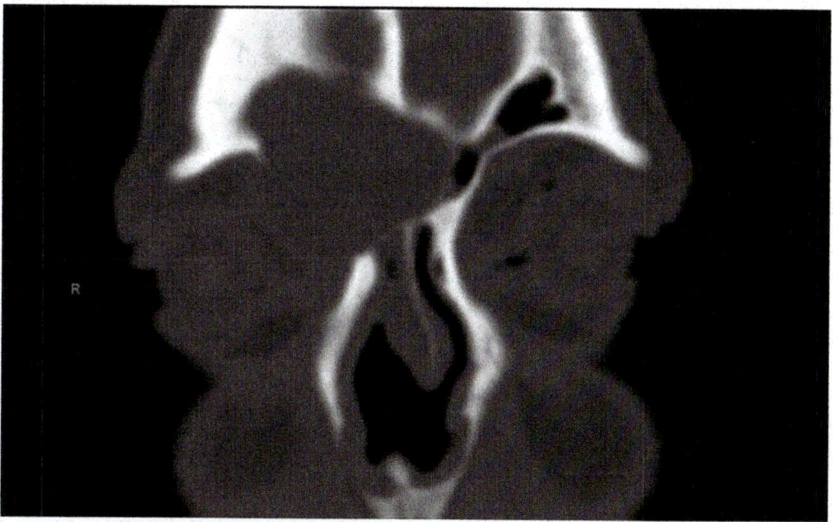

Figure 4.1 Coronal CT scan demonstrating an expansile mass in the right frontal sinus, with inferolateral globe displacement, consistent with a right frontal mucocoele.

- MRI scan:
  - For assessment of neighbouring soft tissue relationship (with intracranial extension)
  - To distinguish from other soft tissue neoplasms
  - Weighted findings depend on water: Protein content, but hypointense on T1 and hyperintense on T2 due to high water content

5. Management:
   - Poorer outcomes associated with delayed pyocoele drainage, posterior ethmoid and sphenoid mucocoeles
   - Management: Usually multi-disciplinary and may involve neurosurgery
     - Conservative: If no deterioration in symptoms, and patient unfit for surgery
     - Medical: Intravenous antibiotics in the event of a mucopyocoele
     - Surgical:
       - ■ Increasing trend for endoscopic drainage with reduced morbidity
       - ■ Previous open approaches not routinely undertaken due to increased morbidity
       - ■ Recurrence in up to 25%
       - ■ Mucopyocoele: Manage with intravenous antibiotics, but if any orbital or IC complications, drain and combine with ESS
6. Differential diagnoses:
   - Sinonasal neoplasm:
     - Benign: Inverted papilloma
     - Malignant: Sinonasal (adenocarcinoma, SCC)

Har-El Classification of Mucocoele (Fronto-Ethmoidal)

Type I:	Frontal (±orbital involvement)
Type II:	Frontal + Ethmoid (±orbital involvement)
Type III:	Posterior table erosion With or without IC involvement (a, b)
Type IV:	Anterior table erosion
Type V:	Posterior + anterior table erosion With or without IC involvement (a, b)

Silent Sinus Syndrome

1. Background:
   - Acquired pathology, also termed imploding maxillary sinus
   - Silent alludes to absence of symptoms
   - Association with smoking
   - Secondary to osteomeatal complex obstruction:
     - Deflected nasal septum
     - Polyps/mucosal disease
     - Concha bullosa/lateralised middle turbinate
     - Presence of infra-orbital air cell (Haller cell)
2. History:
   - Usually, asymptomatic
   - Presentation is diplopia, usually affecting superior and inferior oblique muscles due to attachments to the bony orbit, and thus vulnerability to dysfunction as globe is displaced
   - Hypoesthesia of cheek
3. Examination:
   - Head and neck examination may demonstrate enophthalmos or hypoglobus, facial asymmetry or malar depression
   - Cranial nerve examination to assess acuity and ocular movements
   - Patient may have a pseudo-retraction due to descent of the globe
   - Anterior rhinoscopy/FNE may demonstrate cause for osteomeatal complex obstruction
4. Investigations:
   - CT scan of paranasal sinuses:
     - Abnormal anatomy as a cause of osteomeatal complex obstruction
     - Atelectasis of maxillary sinus
     - Retraction and remodelling of all four walls, with thinning of orbital floor
     - Retraction of uncinate onto inferomedial wall of lamina

5. Management:
   - Conservative:
     - If marginal symptoms and patient preference, can be observed
   - Medical:
     - Usually no role as no underlying medical aetiology
   - Surgical:
     - ESS with large maxillary antrostomy
       - Most symptoms may improve with this intervention alone
       - Key is careful retrograde uncinectomy to avoid orbital perforation
     - Repair of the inferior orbital floor may be necessary
       - Transconjunctival approach
       - Medpore implants
       - Teflon
       - Silicone
6. Differential diagnoses:
   - Chronic sinusitis
   - Trauma (orbital floor fracture)
   - Malignancy of sinus

Inverted Papilloma

1. Background:
   - Benign tumour of the nasal cavity and paranasal sinuses, affecting adults in fifth decade
   - Account for 0.5–1.5% of all nasal neoplasms
   - Male predominance with high rate of recurrence (15–70% due to inadequate clearance)
   - Association with HPV in 40% of cases
   - Predominantly affects lateral nasal wall and maxillary sinus
   - Histologically: Thickened epithelium inverted into underlying connective tissue with an intact basement membrane
   - Malignant conversion (keratinizing and non-keratinizing SCC) in up to 5–15% of cases (figures vary in literature)
   - Synchronous SCC seen in 2% of cases
2. History:
   - Unilateral nasal obstruction
   - Hyposmia
   - Facial pain or headaches due to impaired sinus drainage
   - Epistaxis
   - Epiphora
   - Orbital symptoms or cranial neuropathies in advanced disease/malignant transformation

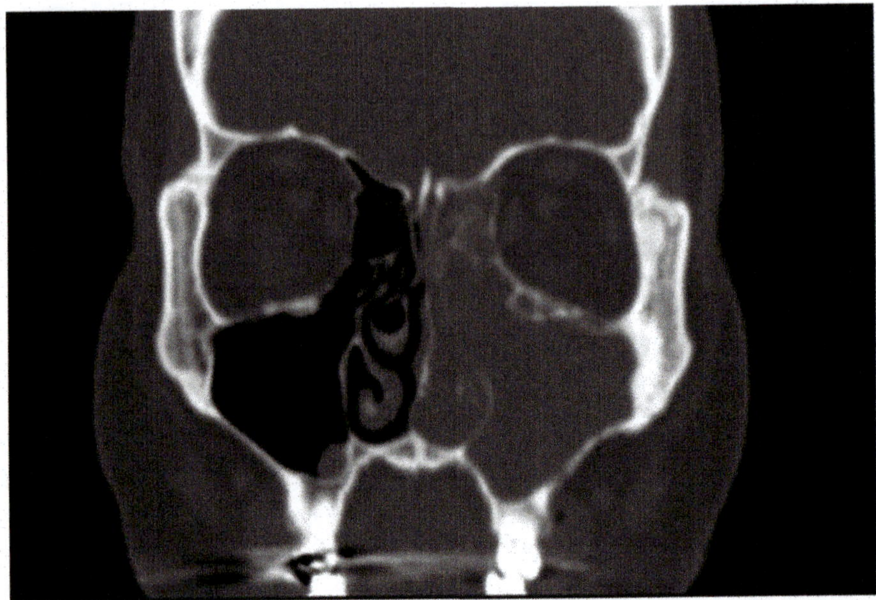

Figure 4.2 Coronal CT scan demonstrating unilateral opacification of the nasal cavity, maxillary and ethmoid sinuses, with some focal hyperostosis. Biopsies confirmed a sinonasal inverted papilloma.

3. Examination:
   - Head and neck examination to rule out nodal disease in event of malignancy, as well as assessment of orbit for proptosis
   - Cranial nerve examination, particularly CN II, III, IV and VI
   - Anterior rhinoscopy/endoscopy may demonstrate abnormal polypoidal tissue within osteomeatal complex
4. Investigations:
   - CT paranasal sinuses:
     - Usually, non-specific soft tissue mass
     - Hyperostosis at site of origin (Figure 4.2)
     - Calcification in 40% of cases
     - Bony resorption
   - MRI paranasal sinuses:
     - Characteristic cerebriform appearance seen on T2 and contrast enhanced T1
5. Management:
   - ESS and complete resection:
     - Medial maxillectomy if involving medial wall/maxillary antrum
     - Resection into subperiosteal plane
     - Drilling of sclerotic bone (origin), to minimise risk of recurrence

   - Post op 5FU may be used
   - Follow-up for 3–5 yrs (Lund and Stammberger)
6. Differential diagnoses:
   - Chronic sinusitis
   - Malignancy of sinus

Evidence:

- Cochrane 2014: Transnasal endoscopic medial maxillectomy in recurrent maxillary sinus inverted papilloma
  - Higher rates of recurrence in Caldwell-Luc vs Endoscopic approach

Krouse classification:

1. Nose lateral nasal wall
2. Ethmoid and maxillary
3. Frontal and sphenoid
4. Beyond confines of nasal cavity/paranasal sinuses OR Malignant transformation

Antrochoanal Polyp

1. Background:
   - Solitary polyps arising from maxillary sinus, with a narrow stalk, extending into nasopharynx
   - Pathologically identical to inflammatory polyps
   - Represent 5% of all nasal polyps (10% adult and 30% paediatric)
   - Slight predominance in males, presenting in third to fifth decade of life
   - Sinusitis present in 25% of patients
2. History:
   - Unilateral nasal obstruction
   - Facial pain or headaches due to impaired sinus drainage
   - Rhinorrhoea and pruritis (although atopic symptoms are rare)
   - Epistaxis
3. Examination:
   - Head and neck examination to rule out nodal disease in event of malignancy due to unilateral nature
     - Larger polyps may extend from nasopharynx into oropharynx
   - Anterior rhinoscopy/FNE to demonstrate unilateral nature
4. Investigations:
   - CT paranasal sinuses: For bony anatomy
     - Mass with mucin density

    - Smooth enlarging of sinus without bony resorption
    - Widening of maxillary accessory ostium
  - MRI paranasal sinuses:
    - Characteristic cerebriform appearance seen on T2 and contrast enhanced T1
5. Management:
  - Usually surgical by means of endoscopic sinus surgery, which has replaced the traditional Caldwell-Luc approach
    - Recurrence rate is reduced by excision of stalk and cuff of adjacent mucosa (7%)
    - Powered instrumentation may minimise risk of recurrence, particularly in revision procedures
6. Differential diagnoses:
  - Glioma
  - Encephalocele
  - JNA
  - Inverted papilloma
  - Mucocoele
  - Sinonasal malignancy
  - Lymphoma

Olfactory Neuroblastoma (Esthesioneuroblastoma)

1. Background:
  - Tumours arising from the basal layer of olfactory epithelium in the superior recess of nasal cavity
  - Neural crest cell origin
  - Usually in anterior ethmoidal cells, extending through cribriform plate into anterior cranial fossa
  - Bi-modal distribution: 20s and then 50s–60s
  - Nodal disease in cervical and retropharyngeal regions seen in 40%
  - Bone is remodelled and resorbed rather than destroyed due to slow growth
  - Can result in Foster-Kennedy syndrome: Optic atrophy and anosmia (unilateral) secondary to frontal lobe mass
2. History:
  - Nasal congestion (70%), timing, length
  - Anosmia (later feature)
  - Blood-stained discharge (50%)
  - Headaches and facial pain
  - Orbital symptoms: Proptosis, epiphora, chemosis, diplopia
  - Cranial nerve symptoms (mainly visual, but hypoesthesia)

3. Examination:
   - Head and neck examination, with nasendoscopy
     - Oropharynx to assess for palatal involvement
     - Assess for nodal disease (25%)
   - Cranial nerve examination including visual assessment
4. Investigations: Identical to sinonasal malignancy:
   - CT: Dumb-bell shape as passing through cribriform plate
   - MRI (orbital and skull base invasion)
   - USS ± FNAC in presence of nodal disease
   - PET-CT if suspected metastases
   - EUA + biopsy
5. Management:
   - MDT discussion
   - Conservative: For patients declining or unfit for medical/surgical intervention
   - Mainstay is surgery:
     - Endoscopic ± open or combined ± Radiotherapy ± Neck dissection
       - Endoscopic surgery contra-indicated if:
       - Orbital exenteration required
       - Skin involvement
       - Optic chiasm involvement
       - ICA/cavernous involvement
       - Large intracranial component
     - Contra-indications:
       - Cavernous sinus/ICA involvement
       - Large intra-cranial component
   - Chemotherapy may be used as a neo-adjuvant treatment or solely for patients not fit for surgery or radiotherapy and also in high Hyams grade tumours
   - Palliative treatment for non-resectable disease
   - Lifelong follow-up with MRI every 3–4 months year 1, 6 monthly for years 2–5, and then 6–9 monthly
     - Follow-up every 6 months lifelong ± EUA and biopsy if suspicion of recurrence
       - 12 monthly after 5 yrs (JLO MD guidelines)
6. Differential diagnoses:
   - Epithelial:
     - Sinonasal SCC/adenocarcinoma
     - SNUC
     - Adenoid cystic carcinoma
     - Malignant melanoma
   - Non-epithelial:
     - Rhabdomyosarcoma
     - T-cell lymphoma
     - Metastatic

Kadish staging and survival outcomes:

A:	Nasal cavity	90% survival at 5 yrs
B:	Paranasal sinuses	70%
C:	Extra-nasal, extra-sinus (oral, orbit, skull base)	50%
D:	Distant metastasis	30%

Nasopharyngeal Malignancy

1. Background:
   - Common site: Fossa of Rosenmuller
   - Risk factors: South-Asian origin (Nitrosamines), EBV, genetic
   - HLA-B17 associated with short-term survival
   - EBV:
     - Early: Intra-cellular antigen (IgA EA)
     - Later: Viral capsule antigen (IgA VCA) – later and most specific finding in NPC
   - Eschelon nodes: Retropharyngeal
2. History:
   - Nasal congestion (timing and length) and blood-stained discharge
   - Headaches or facial pain
   - PMH: Previous sinonasal disease (inverted papilloma), rhinosinusitis
   - Advanced symptoms:
     - Orbital: Proptosis, epiphora
     - Cranial nerve: Diplopia, hypoesthesia
     - Trismus
   - FH: Due to genetic predisposition
3. Examination:
   - Head and neck examination, with flexible nasendoscopy
     - Neck mass: Most common presentation
     - Oropharynx to assess for trismus and palatal involvement
     - Otoscopy: Assess for unilateral glue ear (do not insert grommet as leads to persistent otorrhoea. Consider hearing aid)
   - Cranial nerve examination
4. Investigations:
   - CT (bony landmarks and invasion) and MRI (orbital invasion and distinction from normal tissue as well as carotid artery invasion) in continuity
   - USS ± FNAC in nodal disease
   - PET-CT for advanced disease (T3/T4 as in hypopharyngeal SCC due to likelihood of advanced disease at presentation)

5. Management:
   - Discuss all cases at local MDT
   - Conservative: For patients declining medical/surgical intervention, or poor performance status
   - Mainstay of treatment:
     - Radiotherapy: Nasopharynx + Bilateral necks
     - Concurrent CT: Improves survival in advanced disease by 6%
     - Only indications for surgery:
       - Diagnosis (EUA + biopsy)
       - Recurrent disease (nasopharyngectomy + neck dissection): Re-irradiation is second line

WHO histological classification:

Type I: Keratinising SCC (poor prognosis, less sensitive to RT)
Type II: Non-keratinising SCC (EBV associated, better prognosis, sensitive to RT)
Type III: Undifferentiated (most common, endemic in China, EBV associated, good prognosis, sensitive to RT)

TNM staging in nasopharyngeal malignancy:

T1: Nasopharynx OR nasal cavity OR nasal cavity
T2: Parapharyngeal extension
T3: Sinus, bony erosion of skull base
T4: Intra-cranial, hypopharyngeal, orbital, infra-temporal fossa involvement

N1: Unilateral node ≤6 cm
N2: Bilateral nodal disease ≤6 cm
N3a: ≥6 cm node
N3b: Supraclavicular fossa node

Sinonasal Malignancy

1. Background:
   - Risk factors:
     - Toxins: Chromium, nickel, hydrocarbons (petrol and gas)
       - Woodworkers: Soft wood (SCC), hardwood (adenocarcinoma, more common in ethmoid)
         - Large particles disrupt mucociliary clearance, increasing carcinogen exposure period

    - Textile (leather) and metal (SCC)
    - Radiation
    - Chronic infection
  - Lateral walls, maxillary and ethmoid sinuses as closest proximity to inhaled carcinogen, hence higher incidence
  - Metastasis rare compared to nasopharyngeal
2. History:
  - Unilateral nasal congestion (timing and length) and blood-stained discharge
  - Headaches or facial pain
  - Loose dentition
  - PMH: Previous sinonasal disease (inverted papilloma), rhinosinusitis
  - SH: Occupational exposure to above carcinogens
  - Advanced symptoms:
    - Orbital: Proptosis, epiphora
    - Cranial nerve: Diplopia, hypoesthesia
    - Trismus
3. Examination:
  - Head and neck examination, with flexible nasendoscopy
    - Oropharynx to assess for palatal involvement
    - Assessment of nodal disease
  - Cranial nerve examination:
    - Gottfredson's and Trotter's syndrome
  - Eye examination for proptosis
4. Investigations:
  - CT (bony landmarks and invasion) and MRI (orbital invasion and distinction from normal tissue as well as carotid artery invasion) in continuity
    - Ohngren's line: Medial canthus to angle of mandible. Poorer prognosis if tumour in superior aspect
  - USS ± FNAC if associated adenopathy
  - PET-CT if suspected metastases
  - EUA + biopsy, unless vascular lesion suspected (JIA)
5. Management:
  - MDT involvement
  - Conservative: For patients declining medical/surgical intervention, or unfit
  - Medical:
    - Radiotherapy alone for those not medically fit for surgery
    - Palliative treatment for non-resectable disease
  - Surgical:
    - Mainstay of treatment followed by RT (delivered within 6 weeks of surgery, but high morbidity due to critical structures)
      - Endoscopic:
        - Early stage tumours and some advanced

- Open:
  - Caldwell-Luc
  - Lateral rhinotomy
  - Midfacial degloving
  - Craniofacial resection ± orbital exenteration

- Follow-up with MRI every 3–4 months year 1, 6 monthly for years 2–5, and then 6–9 monthly
- Insufficient evidence to support use of CT. May be used to reduce tumour volume prior to surgery to sensitise tumour to RT

6. Differential diagnoses: As per Esthesioneuroblastoma

Staging:

Maxillary sinus:

T1: Nasal mucosa
T2: Hard palate erosion/middle meatus
T3: Ethmoid sinus, med/inf orbital wall, posterior wall
T4a: Pterygoid plates, cribriform plate, skin, orbit, frontal/sphenoid
T4b: Dura, brain, orbital apex, clivus, nasopharynx, CN (not V2)

Ethmoid sinus:

T1: One subsite, no bony involvement
T2: Two subsites, no bony involvement
T3: Medial orbital wall/floor, maxillary sinus, cribriform plate, pterygoid fossa
T4a: As per maxillary sinus staging
T4b: As per maxillary sinus staging

Rhinophyma

1. Background:
   - Hyperplasia of sebaceous glands histologically
   - Association with Demodex Folliculorum (face mite)
   - Possible housing of occult BCC
   - Lobulated tip may cause nasal obstruction
   - Can be final stage of acne rosacea
     - Not all patients with rhinophyma will have acne rosacea
     - Rosacea (F > M)
     - Rhinophyma (M is 30× > F)
   - Caucasian males affected in fifth and sixth decades of life
   - No association with alcohol or facial flushing
   - Early signs: Dilated pores and telangiectasia

2. History:
   - Timing
   - Onset
   - Specific regions with rapid changes/ulceration
   - Nasal obstruction/functional impairment
   - Psychological impact of condition
3. Examination:
   - External nasal examination
   - Assessment of telangiectasia, dilated pores, isolated lesions (BCC)
   - Anterior rhinoscopy and dynamic assessment (external valve collapse)
4. Investigations:
   - Only indication would be histology in suspected occult BCC
5. Management:
   - Conservative:
     - Skin cleansing
   - Medical:
     - Benzoyl peroxide
     - Antibiotics (Tetracyclines are bacteriostatic as well as anti-inflammatory)
     - Retinoids (isotretinoin – teratogenic)
   - Surgical: Array of modalities described
     - Aims:
       - Debulk
       - Re-contour
       - Haemostasis
       - Prevent post-operative complications
     - Modalities: Usually combination of below:
       - Excisional: Allows histopathological evaluation:
         - Excision with graft (colour mismatch means grafts are rarely utilised)
         - Partial thickness: Preserves sebaceous glands (not including reticular layer of dermis when excising)
         - Dermabrasion: Utilised as adjunct for contouring
       - Ablative:
         - Loop diathermy excision
         - Coblation
       - Laser:
         - Argon, CO_2 or KTP

Epiphora

1. Background:
   - Excessive tearing and overflow

- As a result of:
    - Excessive production:
        - Bacterial infection (dacryocystitis, blepharitis)
        - Inflammation (GPA, Sjogren's, SLE)
        - Trauma
        - Aberrant nerve regeneration following cranial nerve VII palsy
        - Allergic pathology
    - Inadequate/impaired drainage:
        - Previous trauma (facial fractures)
        - Iatrogenic (previous ocular or endoscopic sinus surgery resulting in blockage of Hasner's valve)
        - Obstructive due to lacrimal sac tumour

2. History:
    - Timing, onset of duration and side affected
    - Seasonal variation/allergic symptoms
    - Mucoid discharge (conjunctivitis)
    - Association with gustation (aberrant regeneration)
    - Visual symptoms (keratitis)
    - PMH: Trauma, surgery, radiotherapy
    - DH: Pilocarpine, chemotherapy
3. Examination:
    - Examination of face to assess for scars
    - Eye examination:
        - Obstructive masses in medial canthus (lacrimal sac tumour)
        - Erythema, conjunctivitis or pus expressed
        - Entropion/ectropion
    - Evidence of synkinesis
    - Flexible nasendoscopy to assess inferior meatus, for masses, crusting or polyps
4. Investigations:
    - Schirmer's test
    - Fluorescein dye disappearance test
    - Dacrocystography
    - MRI/CT if suspected neoplastic cause
5. Management:
    - Dependent on aetiology:
    - Medical:
        - Lacrilube/viscotears
        - Topical therapy for infective causes (conjunctivitis)
        - Surgical:
            - Punctoplasty (widening by incising punctal opening)
            - Balloon dilatation of strictures

- DCR (endoscopic 85% success vs external 92% success):
  - Dilatation of superior and inferior canaliculi with probe
  - Infiltration with Lignospan
  - Maxillary line identified (medial projection of the frontal process of maxilla – axilla to root of inferior turbinate)
  - Fundus of lacrimal sac is usually 10 mm above axilla of MT
  - Inferior limit is usually half-way along the maxillary line
  - Mucosal flap created over lacrimal bone
  - Cannulation with lacrimal light pipe do confirm positioning of lacrimal sac
  - Diamond drill ± Kerrison's punch forceps to expose lacrimal sac
  - Vertical incision into lacrimal sac
  - Crawford stents are inserted through superior and inferior canaliculi, a further sheath is passed over stents and clipped intra-nasally to prevent extrusion
    - No high-level evidence to suggest benefit of stents
  - Flaps are positioned superiorly and inferiorly with overlying Surgicel
  - Mitomycin may be used for reduction in granulation tissue formation

Pinnaplasty/Otoplasty

1. Background:
   - Common auricular defects:
     - Prominauris: Increase in auriculocephalic angle due to underdevelopment of antihelical fold
     - Cryptotia: Underdeveloped scapha and anti-helical crura (upper ear buried below skin)
     - Cup ear: Folded helical rim
   - Common conditions with ear deformities: All first and second arch anomalies
     - Treacher-Collins
     - Goldenhar syndrome
     - Hemifacial microsomia
   - Normal auriculocephalic angle = 30 degrees. Prominauris is >40 degrees
   - Normal height (vertical) = 6 cm
   - 85% of adult ear size reached by 6 yrs
2. History:
   - Parental concerns raised before patient
   - Always explore impact of condition on patient

    - Patient likely to report bullying when entering secondary education
    - Will report low confidence levels and mood
    - Hampered school performance
  - PMH:
    - First arch anomalies as above
    - Cardiac (CHARGE), renal or genital abnormalities (BORS and CHARGE)
3. Examination:
  - Evaluate components:
    - Helix
    - Anti-helix
    - Tragus
    - Anti-tragus
    - Scaphoid and triangular fossae
    - Lobule
  - Evaluate for other abnormalities: Branchial arch anomalies, clefts
4. Management:
  - MDT: Clinical psychology input is helpful
  - Conservative:
    - No intervention and observation
    - Taping ears
    - Psychotherapy
    - EarWell cradle (within 1 week, re-shapes ear using adhesive anchoring)
  - Surgical: Dependent on local funding
    - Techniques:
      - Mustarde: Horizontal mattress sutures posteriorly to create antihelical fold. Mattress 2 mm apart, 1-cm width, 4.0 undyed Prolene or Ethibond (Figure 4.3)
      - Sculpturing (Weerda): Scoring or thinning to weaken cartilage and create convexity for the anti-helical fold (Figure 4.4)
      - Farrior technique: Combination of above
      - Furnass technique: Concha setback by suturing concha to mastoid periosteum. Has replaced Mustard technique
      - Earfold device: Nickel-titanium implant under local anaesthetic (visible if thin skinned)
    - Complications:
      - Most common complaint is under-correction/unhappy aesthetic outcome
      - Infection (perichondritis) and skin necrosis as complications are rare
      - Scarring (keloid)
      - Hypoesthesia

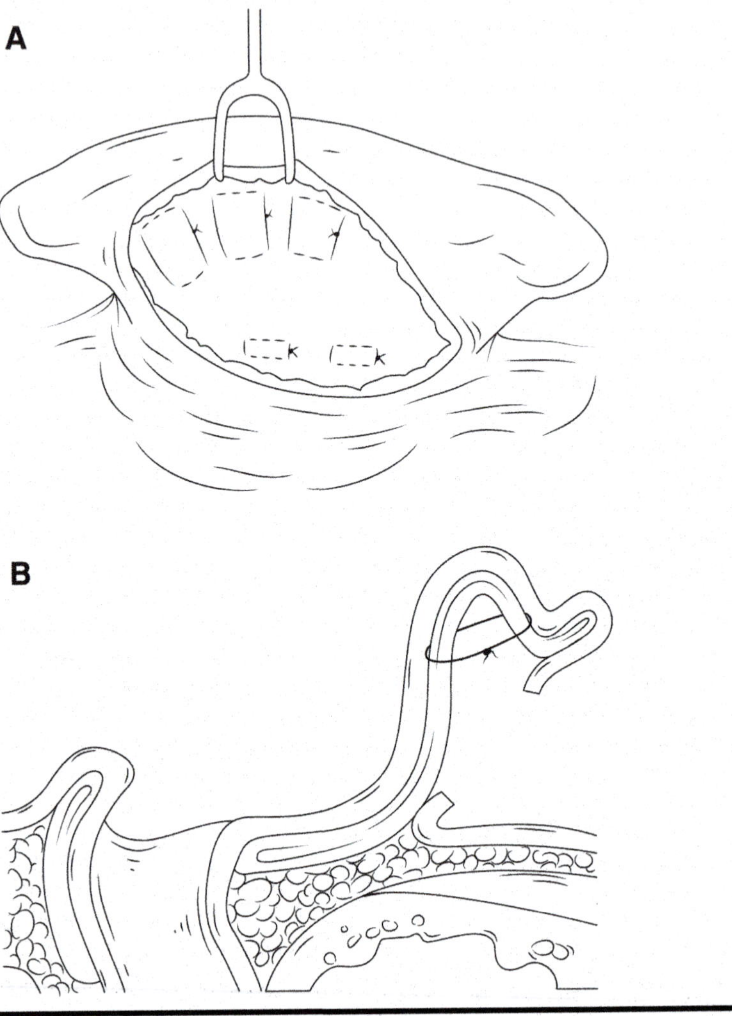

Figure 4.3 Mustarde otoplasty suture technique. (a) Posterior and (b) axial views demonstrating suture technique.

- Telephone ear deformity: Overcorrection of middle 1/3 of ear
- Reverse telephone ear deformity is under correction of middle 1/3, or over correction of upper and lower 1/3

- Post-operative management (varies between units):
  - 7 days antibiotics (co-amoxiclav)
  - Head bandage down 5–7 days
  - Headband 3 months nocte

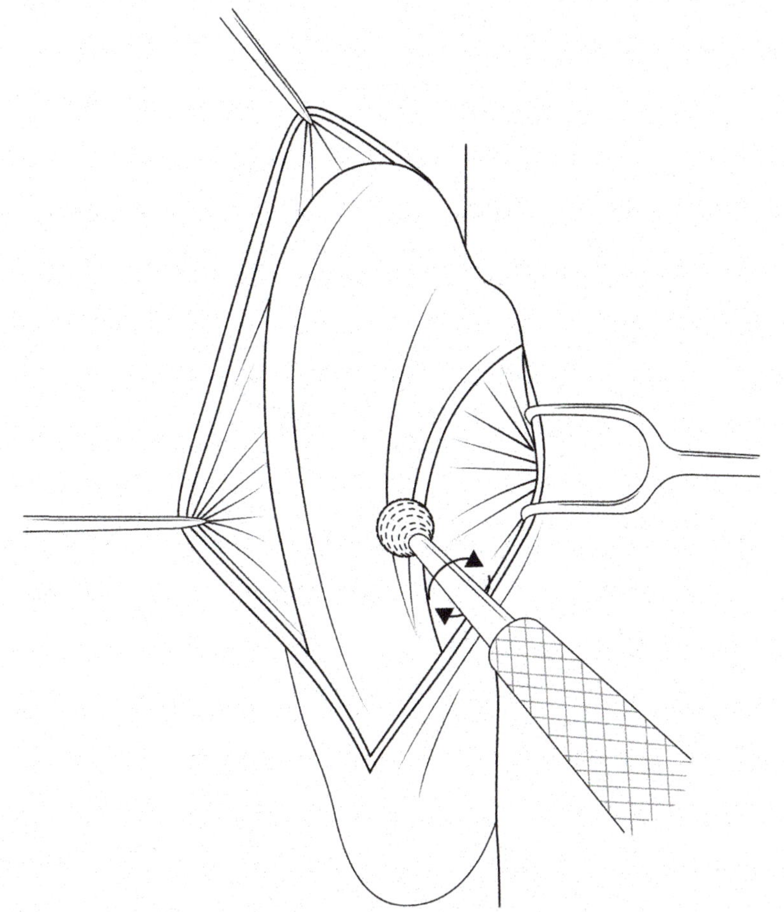

Figure 4.4 Weerda cartilage scoring/thinning technique.

Facial Plastics

- Reconstructive ladder:
  - Secondary healing
  - Primary closure
  - Grafts (STSG, FTSG)
    - STSG: Contains epidermis and some dermis
    - FTSG: Contains entire epidermis and dermis (post-aural, pre-auricular, supraclavicular). Blood supply derived through:
      - Imbibition: Nutrition from underlying bed = 1–2 days
      - Inosculation: Small vessels from graft meeting vessels in bed = Day 2
      - Angiogenesis: Neovascularisation = 4–7 days

- Local flap (rotation, advancement)
- Tissue expansion
- Regional flap (pec major, latissimus dorsi)
- Free flap (radial forearm, antero-lateral thigh, fibular)
- Prosthesis

■ Skin closure:
- Elliptical closure/fusiform closure requires <30 degrees, otherwise consider graft or M-plasty. Length to width ratio of 3:1
- Scars should ideally be placed at junction of facial aesthetic units
- Closure should be along axis of relaxed skin tension line (RSTL)
    - RSTLs are parallel to wrinkles and perpendicular to contraction of muscles
    - Langer's lines are perpendicular to RSTL
    - LME is a plane with least tension during closure – perpendicular to RSTL
- Scar cosmesis:
    - Z-plasty lengthens and re-distributes force and aligns scar along RSTL or aesthetic subunit junction (optimal position):
        - ■ 60 degrees = 75%
        - ■ 45 degrees = 50%
        - ■ 30 degrees = 25%
    - W-plasty: Along RSTL, 6 mm limbs at 60 degrees and geometric broken lines (>45 degrees to RSTL)

■ Flaps:
- Based on tissue: Cutaneous (skin with superficial fascia), fasciocutaneous (skin and deep fascia), myocutaneous (fasciocutaneous + muscle) or visceral (colon, jejunum, omentum)
- Based on vasculature: Axial (named artery/vein, parallel to skin surface) or random (vasculature perpendicular to skin surface)
- Based on donor site (local, regional or free): See Table 4.3

Layers of skin:

■ Epidermis: Stratum basalis, spinosum, granulosum, lucidum and corneum

■ Dermis:
- Reticular layer: Basal layer, dense connective tissue, sebaceous glands, nerves, hair follicles
- Papillary layer: Loose connective tissue, vessels and nerves

■ Hypodermis (subcutaneous)

Table 4.3 Flaps Based on Donor Site

Local Flaps (Adjacent Tissue)			
Type	***Name***	***Blood Supply***	***Properties***
Advancement (Linear movement)	H (Figure 4.5) V-Y T-Plasty	Random pattern	
Rotation (Around pivot point)	Hatchet/double hatchet (Figure 4.8)	Random pattern	
Transposition (Lifted and orientated)	Limberg (Figure 4.6) Bi-lobed (double transposition) (Figure 4.7)	Random pattern	
Interpolated (Rests on bridge of tissue)	Paramedian forehead flap (Figure 4.9) Cheek flap	Supratrochlear artery Angular artery	
Regional Flaps			
Name	***Type***	***Blood Supply***	***Properties***
Pectoralis major	Cutaneous or myocutaneous	Thoracoacromial artery (pectoral branch)	Pharyngeal defects, salvage surgery
Trapezius	Myocutaneous	Occipital, transverse cervical and dorsal scapular arteries	Limited arc of rotation and increased donor morbidity
Latissimus dorsi	Myocutaneous	Thoracodorsal artery	
Deltopectoral	Fasciocutaneous	Perforating vessels of internal mammary artery	Oral cavity oropharyngeal, hypopharyngeal defects
Sternocleidomastoid	Myocutaneous	Segmental: Occipital, post-auricular, transverse cervical and superior thyroid arteries	

(Continued)

Table 4.3 Flaps Based on Donor Site ***(Continued)***

Free Flaps (Osseous)			
Name	***Type***	***Blood Supply***	***Properties***
Radial Forearm	Fascio or osseocutaneous	Radial artery	Tubed flap in pharyngeal reconstruction or floor of mouth
Scapular	Osseocutaneous	Circrumflex scapular artery	Facial, mandibular defects
Fibula	Osseocutaneous	Peroneal artery	Mandibular reconstruction
Iliac Crest (DCIA flap)	Osteomyocutaneous	Deep circumflex iliac artery	
Free Flaps (Soft Tissue)			
Name	***Type***	***Blood Supply***	***Properties***
Rectus abdominis	Myocutaneous	Inferior and superior epigastric arteries	Orbit, maxilla and skull base use
Anterolateral thigh (ALT)	Fasciocutaneous	Lateral circumflex femoral artery	
Jejunum	Visceral	Superior mesenteric arcade	Used in circumferential pharyngeal defect
Gracilis	Muscle flap	Profunda femoris	Facial reanimation

Scars

1. Background:
   - Keloids and hypertrophic scars most likely secondary to local, hormonal and genetic factors
   - Described as variations of normal wound healing

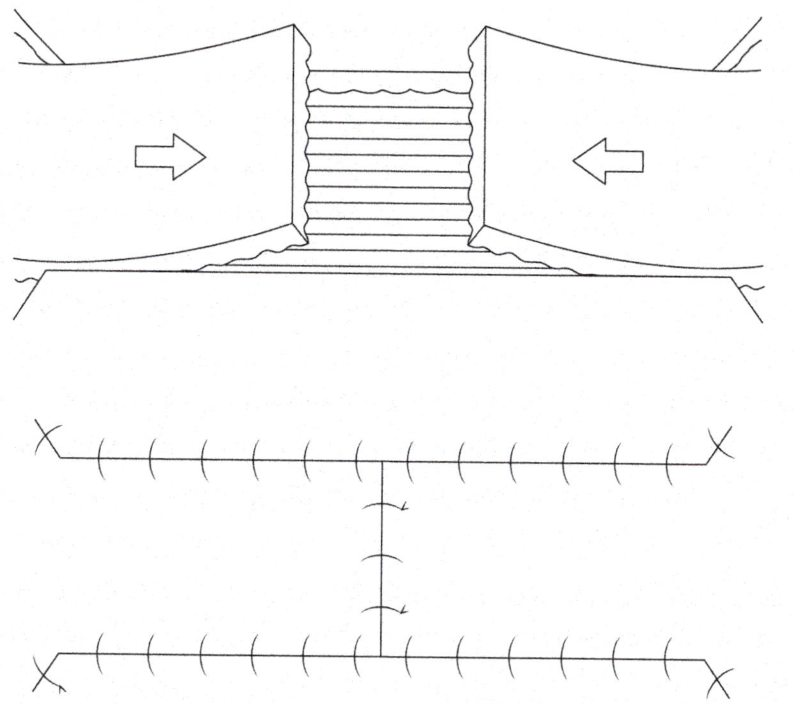

Figure 4.5 H-advancement flap.

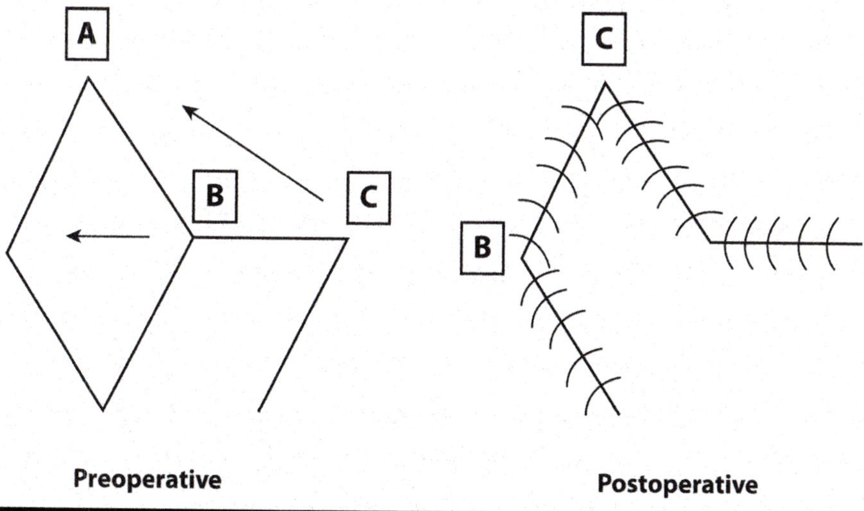

Figure 4.6 Limberg transposition flap.

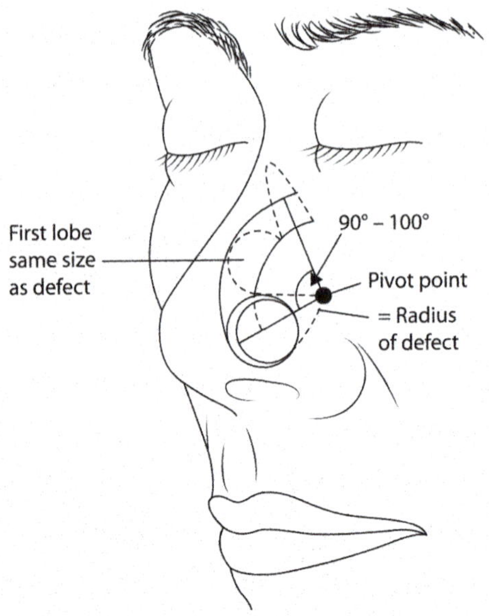

Figure 4.7 Bi-lobed, double transposition flap.

- Keloid scar:
  - Increased incidence in Afro-Caribbean population
  - Excessive random deposition of type 3 collagen, replaced by type 1
  - Associated with wounds with greater tension
- Hypertrophic scar:
  - Excess scar formation
  - Flattens with time

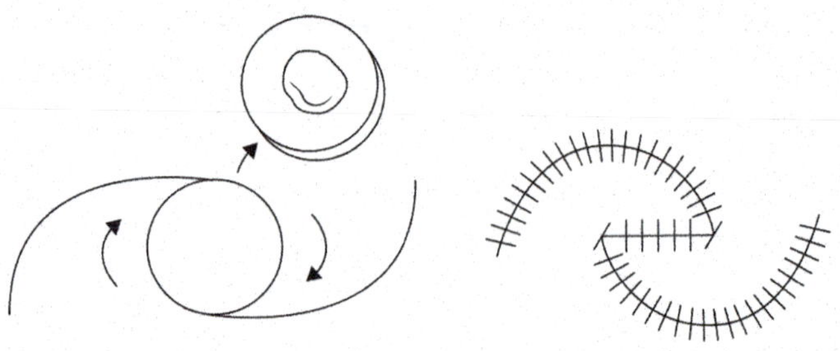

Figure 4.8 Double hatchet rotation flap.

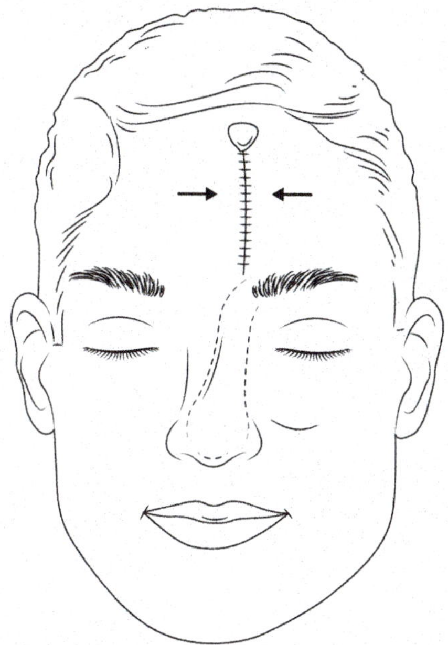

Figure 4.9 Paramedian forehead interpolated flap.

	Keloid	*Hypertrophic*
Incidence	Rare	Common
Timing (onset)	Soon after injury	Delayed
Progression	Increased with time	Flattening with time
Skin colour	Dark skin associated	No association with colour
Genetic predisposition	Yes	Unknown
Symptoms	Painful and itchy	Usually asymptomatic
Boundaries	Beyond margin	Within margin
Collagen arrangement	Random	Parallel
Steroid response	Marginal	Good/complete
Location	Sternum, deltoid earlobe	Skin over flexor surfaces
Recurrence	Yes	Unlikely

2. History:
   - History of local trauma (skin piercings)
   - Pain
   - Duration of symptoms and progression over time is key
   - PMH: Previous surgery
   - FH: Keloids
3. Examination:
   - Location is usually key and will indicate likely pathology
   - Examine confines of lesion
4. Management: Mainly keloids
   - Conservative:
     - Avoid surgery
       - Tension free closure and parallel to RSTL or in creases
       - Use fine suture material and remove early
     - Pressure dressings
     - Sun protection
   - Medical:
     - Moisturising
     - Silicone patches/gel
     - Steroid (Triamcinolone):
       - 40 mg/mL
       - Two to three injections 1/12 apart, max 6
       - First-line therapy for keloids
       - Inhibits fibroblast activity and collagen synthesis
       - Increases collagenase production
     - Radiotherapy: ONLY if benefits outweigh risks
     - 5-FU
     - Laser (ablative)
   - Intralesional excision + steroid: Multi-modality treatment is associated with less risk of recurrence in keloids
5. Differential diagnoses:
   - Dermatofibroma

Stages of wound healing:

- Three stages:
  - Inflammatory:
    - Haemostasis:
      - TXA2 mediated vasoconstriction, then vasodilation (Histamine, NO)
      - Endothelial wall contraction, collagen visible
      - Platelet plug formation

- Inflammation:
  - Neutrophil migration within 4–6 hrs
  - Macrophage migration up to 48 hrs
  - Fibroblast migration at 48 hrs produce collagen and elastin
- Proliferative:
  - Epithelialisation
  - Neovascularisation: Granulation tissue + Angiogenes (VEGF mediated)
  - Collagen deposition: Type III, then type I
  - Wound contraction: Myofibroblast mediated
- Remodeling:
  - Increase in type I collagen, increase in tensile strength, with fibres now parallel
- Maximal tensile strength at 6 months, and usually 80% of original strength

Evidence:

- Cochrane Collaborative (2013): Silicone gel sheeting for preventing the development of hypertrophic and keloid scars and for treating existing hypertrophic and keloid scars
  - Weak evidence for silicone sheeting

Cutaneous Basal Cell Carcinoma

1. Background:
   - Basal cell carcinoma (BCC) most common skin cancer
     - Nodular: Rolled pearly edges, central ulceration, telangiectasia (lowest risk)
     - Superficial: Rare and resembles psoriasis or eczema
     - Pigmented: As with nodular, but darkened colour
     - Morphoeic: Ill-defined, scar like (high-risk)
   - High-risk features: >2 cm, central face/H-zone, immunosuppression, indistinct margins (morphoeic)
   - Multiple actinic keratosis/solar keratosis: Pre-malignant, risk factor for BCC, UV damaged skin, seen in elderly
2. History:
   - Duration, site, size
   - Risk factors: UV light, fair skin, sun exposure, immunosuppression, radiotherapy
   - PMH: Previous skin cancers, Gorlin Goltz syndrome (BCC, keratogenic cysts, bifid ribs, cerebral calcification), radiation exposure

- Social history: Occupational sun exposure

3. Examination:
   - Fitzpatrick skin type
   - A(symmetry), B(order), C(olour, 2+ lesions), D(iameter, >6 mm), E(levation)/ Edges (rolled, pearly, irregular) and ulceration
   - Full head and neck examination: Lymphadenopathy, parotid deposits of SCC, facial nerve function
4. Investigations:
   - US guided FNAC for suspicious nodes, and resection if negative but high suspicion
   - No imaging required in N0 disease
     - CT for bony invasion
     - MRI for perineural invasion (facial palsy)
   - Punch biopsy (4 mm) preferred for diagnosis (or incisional): Especially in cosmetically sensitive areas. Biopsy in peripheries with no ulceration to prevent diagnosis of acellular material
5. Management:
   - Medical:
     - Photodynamic therapy for superficial BCC
     - Excisional curettage: <1 cm and low-risk lesions
     - Cryotherapy: <4 mm and low-risk lesions i.e. superficial
     - 5% imiquimod
   - Surgery:
     - Excision with 4–5 mm margins
       - 3 mm gives 85% clearance
       - 4–5 mm gives 95% clearance
       - 3 mm in cosmetically sensitive areas if reconstructive options limited
       - In the absence of MOHS facilities, up to 1.5cm margin for confirmed morphoeic BCC
       - British association of dermatologists: Delayed reconstruction recommended in all histologically unconfirmed lesions, even if index of suspicion is low
     - MOHS:
       - 97% 5 yr survival
       - 95% 5 yr survival in recurrence
       - Indications:
         - Recurrence
         - High-risk areas: H-zone
         - Cosmetically sensitive areas
         - High-risk lesions
     - Radiotherapy:
       - Electron beam RT

    - Elderly and frail not fit for surgery
- Vismodegib monoclonal treatment:
    - Locally advanced metastatic BCC
    - Not amenable to surgery
    - Gorlin Goltz syndrome
- Follow up:
    - High-risk incompletely excised: Re-excise 5–10 mm margins
    - Completely excised: Discharge after 1 FU
    - Multiple: Annual review

Cutaneous Squamous Cell Carcinoma

1. Background:
   - Second most common cutaneous malignancy
   - 1–4% metastatic potential
   - High-risk features: >2 cm, immunosuppression, >2 mm deep, Clark level 4, poorly/undifferentiated, perineural invasion, H-zone of face (see figure 4.10)
   - Actinic keratosis: Thick, crusting skin on scalp in elderly patients
     - Solar damage; premalignant = 10% of progression to SCC
2. History: As per BCC
3. Examination: As per BCC
4. Investigations: Largely identical to BCC, except:

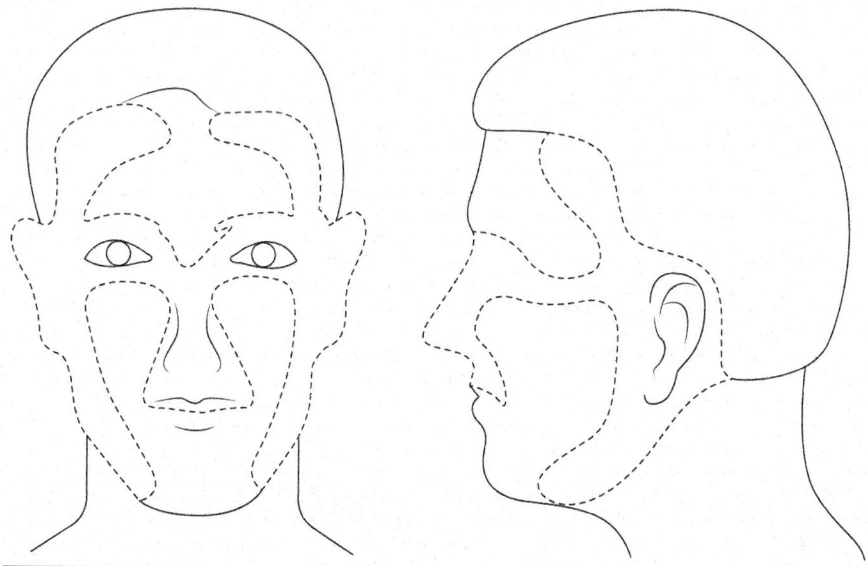

Figure 4.10 H-Zone of face in relation to high-risk cutaneous malignancy.

- CT neck/chest if:
  - Parotid involvement
  - N+ disease
  - Perineural or bony invasion (consider MRI)

5. Management:
   - Surgery:
     - 4 mm margin in low-risk lesions: 95% clearance
     - 6 mm in high-risk lesions
     - Neck dissection + parotidectomy in clinically positive nodal disease
       - P+N0: Superficial parotidectomy + levels I–III
       - P+N+: Superficial parotidectomy + levels I–III (+V if clinically involved)
       - P0N+:
         - Anterior to tragus: Levels I–IV
         - Posterior to tragus: Levels II–V
       - Post-operative RT:
         - Positive margins
         - >N1 disease
         - Extracapsular spread
         - Perineural or lymphovascular invasion
     - MOHS: Indications as per BCC
     - Radiotherapy:
       - Cosmetically sensitive areas
       - Unfit for surgery
     - Surveillance in SCC:
       - Low-risk SCC: Discharge after single FU
       - High-risk SCC: FU 6 monthly for 2 yrs
       - High-risk SCC: Incompletely excised – re-excise

T staging:

T1: <2 cm and <2 high-risk factors
T2: >2 cm or 2 high-risk factors
T3: Bony invasion
T4: Perineural or skull base involvement

Malignant Melanoma

1. Background:
   - Linked to UV exposure
   - 50% have BRAF gene mutation

- Worse prognosis: BANS (scalp and ear have significantly worse prognosis than neck and face)
  - Back (upper)
  - Arms
  - Neck
  - Scalp
- Mucosal melanomas start at T3 staging and present with epistaxis or nasal congestion
  - Management is surgical excision with clear margins where possible
- Types:
  - Superficial spreading: Most common. Irregular asymmetric margins. Radial followed by vertical growth
  - Nodular: Worst prognosis. Grows aggressively in vertical direction. Bleeding and ulceration tendency
  - Lentigo maligna melanoma: Spreads along dermo-epidermal junction. Seen in older patients with sun damaged skin
  - Acral lentiginous: Soles or hands and feet. Seen in African and Asian population

2. History: Largely identical to BCC and SCC
   - Family history
3. Examination: As per BCC and SCC
4. Investigations:
   - Staging imaging for regional or distant metastasis (high-risk groups)
   - MRI brain in stage 4 disease
   - Sentinel node biopsy if lesions >0.75 mm
   - N+ disease investigated with FNA/core biopsy
   - Serum LDH: Influences staging
   - Excisional biopsy treatment of choice with subdermal fat included: 2–5 mm margin
   - Punch biopsy in large or cosmetically sensitive area (2–4 mm punch at thickest site of lesion)
5. Management:
   - Surgery:

Depth	Excision margin
Melanoma in situ:	5 mm margin
Up to 1 mm:	1 cm margin
1.01–2 mm:	1–2 cm margin
2.01–4 mm	2–3 cm margin
>4 mm	2–3 cm margin

- Vemurafenib monoclonal treatment:
  - In BRAF gene mutations
  - Advanced disease
- Stereotactic RT: Metastatic disease i.e. brain

Risk factors:

- Fair skin
- UV light exposure
- Multiple naevi
- Family history
- Immunosuppression
- Familial dysplastic naevus syndrome: 50% risk by 50 yrs age

TNM staging:

T1: ≤1 mm
T2: 1.01–2.0 mm
T3: 2.01–4.0 mm
T4: >4 mm

All T stages have a or b based on ulceration

N1: 1 node
N2: 2–3 nodes
N3: >4 nodes

M1a: Skin or distant LN
M1b: Lung involvement
M1c Viscera + LDH elevated

Mucosal melanoma:

T3: Mucosa only
T4a: Soft tissue, cartilage, bone
T4b: Intracranial, carotid, cranial nerve involvement

N0: No nodes
N1: Regional nodes

Topical Therapies in Rhinology

Flixonase:	Fluticasone propionate
Avamys:	Fluticasone furoate
Betnesol:	Betamethasone sodium phosphate
Rinatec:	Ipratropium bromide

Dymista:	Azelastine hydrochloride + fluticasone propionate
Rhinocort:	Budesonide
Co-phenylcaine:	Lignocaine 5% + phenylephrine 0.5%
Naseptin:	Neomycin sulphate + chlorhexidine dihydrochloride (Arachis oil content)

Chapter 5

Examination Stations

Adnan Darr, Karan Jolly, Keshav K. Gupta and Jameel Muzaffar

Contents

Introduction

As part of the FRCS (ORL-HNS) viva, you will be required to perform multiple examinations. This chapter will discuss the framework to approach the four main ENT examinations: otology, rhinology, head and neck (including thyroid) and cranial nerves. As for all clinical examinations, it is paramount to be aware the patient in front of you may be more used to experiencing a medical examination than others. This aspect of the Part B examination constitutes 20% of the total mark (5% per station).

It is important to make a conscious effort to make your patient feel comfortable. This starts with a formal introduction in all cases before commencing. Most clinical examinations in ENT follow the same stepwise approach: Introduction, general inspection, palpation, instrumentation, special tests and conclusion. The introductory aspect will assume all candidates are bare below the elbows, have washed their hands appropriately, and have proceeded to introduce themselves. Proceed to ask the patient their name, how they would like to be addressed and gain consent by briefly explaining what the examination will entail. Ask if they have any concerns, or pain, and commence on the contra-lateral side.

DOI: 10.1201/9781003247098-5

Otology

1. Introduction:
   - Introduce yourself by name and role
   - Confirm the patient's details (name and date of birth)
   - Explain the steps of examination you are planning to undertake
   - Empower the patient to ask questions or stop you at any time
   - Confirm that the patient consents for you to proceed
2. Inspection: Frontal and lateral views
   - Pinna deformities: Microtia or prominauris
   - Mastoid: Surgical scars, swelling, erythema
   - Skin: Pits, sinuses, tags, evidence of cellulitis
   - Comparison with contralateral side
3. Palpation
   - Pre- and post-auricular lymphadenopathy
   - Tragal/pinna tenderness
   - Mastoid tenderness and/or swelling
4. Otoscopy:
   - Pull pinna postero-superiorly to straighten EAC
   - Mastoid cavity:
     - Infection, wax, cholesteatoma and discharge
     - Causes of discharge in pre-existing mastoid cavity:
       - Inadequate saucerisation
       - Large cavity
       - High facial ridge
       - Disease recurrence
       - Perforation
       - Inadequate meatoplasty
   - EAC: Swelling, flaking (eczema), discharge, debris, blood, masses (granulation, exostoses, osteomas)
   - TM (Figure 5.1):
     - Quadrant assessment:
       - Light reflex/cone of light, colour, perforation, tympanosclerosis, fluid level, masses, infection, retraction
5. Special tests: Four Fs
   - **F**ree field testing: At 2 distances (15 and 60 cm) with gross masking of contralateral ear (tragal rub)
     - 2/3 words correct is a pass
     - Approximate conversion to dB summarised in boxed text
   - **F**orks: Rinne's and Weber's tests (summarised in boxed text)
     - Use 512 Hz tuning fork: Best tone decay, less overtones, less vibratory tactile sensation

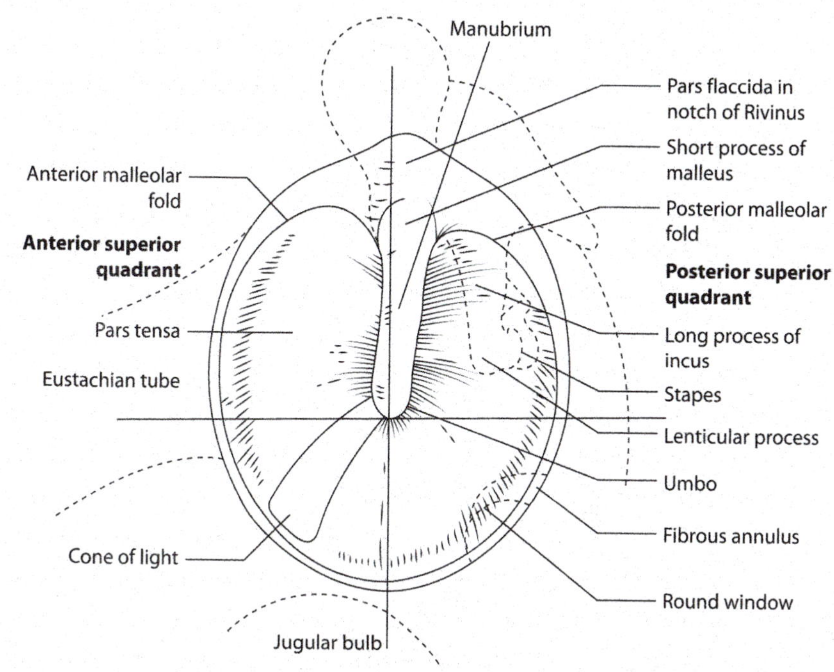

Figure 5.1 Tympanic membrane quadrants and anatomy.

- Rinne's test:
  - Place fork 2 cm in front of EAC (position A) and then place on mastoid process (position B)
  - Ask patient if loudest in position A or B
  - Rinne positive = AC > BC which is either normal or SNHL
  - Rinne negative = BC > AC which is conductive HL
- Weber's test:
  - Place fork along vertex or chin
  - Ask patient in which ear they hear the sound the loudest, or if equal on both sides
  - Equal = normal or bilateral hearing loss
  - Localised to one side = towards conductive HL or away from SNHL

– Fistula test:
- Application of intermittent pressure to tragus can elicit nystagmus
- Negative: Normal
- True positive: Superior SCC dehiscence, horizontal SCC erosion, round window rupture

    - False negative: Cholesteatoma covering fistula, dead labyrinth
    - False positive: Congenital syphilis (hypermobile stapes), Meniere's disease (stapes connected to utricular macula by fibrous bands)
  - Facial nerve assessment:
6. Conclusion:
  - Thank the patient and ask if they have any questions
  - Relay to the examiner that you would complete your examination by undertaking:
    - A full head and neck examination for adenopathy
    - FNE to assess the post-nasal space for any masses in the context of a unilateral middle ear effusion
    - Cranial nerve assessment: V, VI (petrous apex) and IX, X, XI (jugular foramen)
    - Formal hearing tests: Pure tone audiometry, tympanometry

Approximate conversion of free field hearing test to dB and degree of hearing loss

Volume of Voice	*Distance (cm)*	*Approximate Conversion*
Whisper	15	Normal hearing (<12 dB)
	60	Mild hearing loss (<34 dB)
Conversational	15	Mild-moderate hearing (<48 dB)
	60	Moderate hearing loss (<56 dB)
Loud	15	Severe hearing loss (<76 dB)
	60	Profound hearing loss (<90 dB)

Interpretation of Weber's and Rinne's tuning fork tests.

Hearing Loss	*Rinne's Test*	*Weber's Test*
None	AC > BC	Midline/no lateralisation
SNHL	AC > BC (bilaterally)	Lateralised to normal ear
CHL	BC > AC	Lateralised to affected ear

Rhinology

1. Introduction:
  - Introduce yourself by name and role

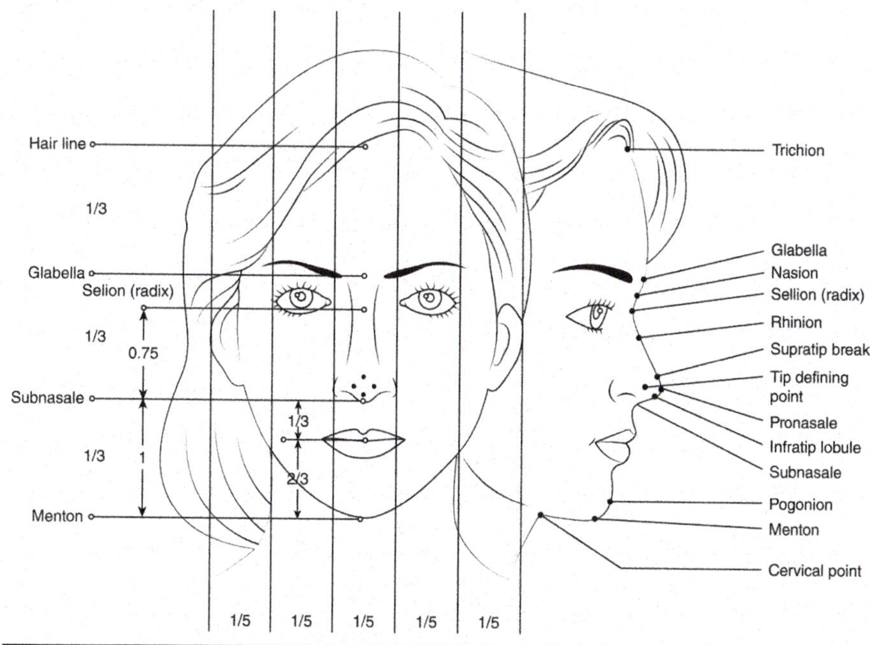

Figure 5.2 Facial landmarks.

- Confirm the patient's details (name and date of birth)
- Explain the steps of examination you are planning to undertake
- Empower the patient to ask questions or stop you at any time
- Confirm that the patient consents for you to proceed

2. Inspection: Frontal, lateral, basal, plan and oblique views
    - Scars: Inverted V, lateral rhinotomy, Lynch-Howarth
    - Deformities: C shape, S shape, skew, saddle nose, pollybeak
        - Frontal view: Figure 5.2
            - Horizontal thirds
            - Vertical fifths
            - Brow-tip aesthetic line: Curvilinear line from medial along lateral nasal wall tip should be undisrupted
            - Assessment of nasal bone symmetry and nasal tip (definition points and bulbosity)
        - Lateral view
            - Nasion: Nasofrontal suture, sellion (deepest point of nasofrontal angle), radix (sellion and nasion)
            - Nasal bone assessment: Dorsal hump, pseudo hump, saddle deformity, pollybeak
            - Tip assessment: Pollybeak (prominence of supratip)

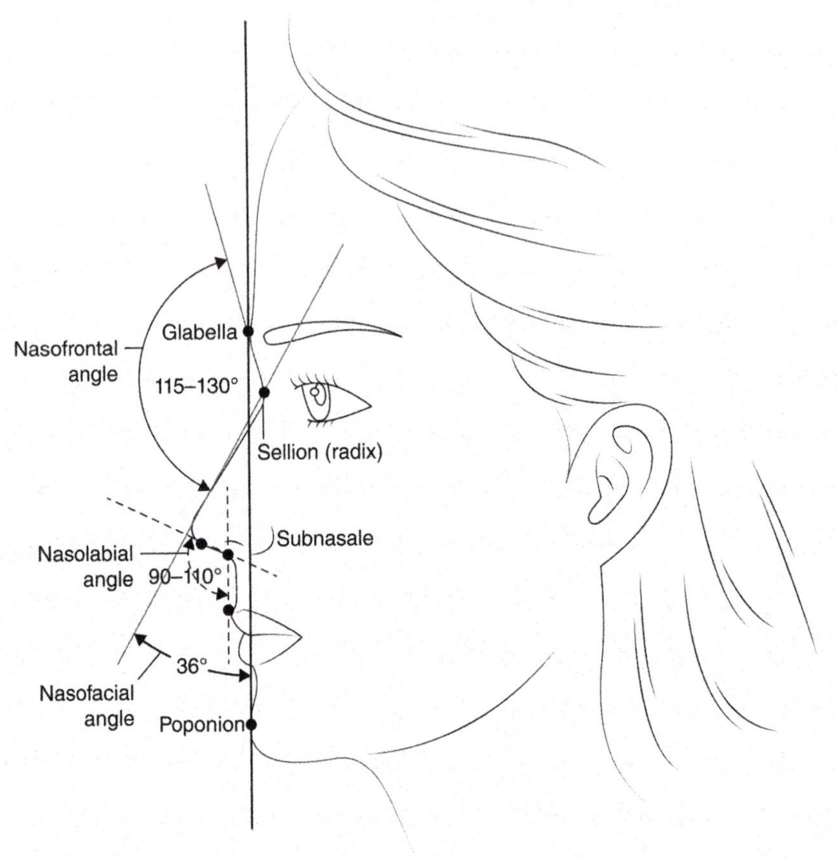

Figure 5.3 Facial angles.

- ■ Angles/measurements: Figure 5.3
  - o Tip projection: Normal 0.6× radix to tip
  - o Tip rotation: Normal nasolabial angle 90° male, 100° female
  - o Nasofrontal angle: Normal 110–120° male, 120–130° female
  - o Columella: Normal show 2–4 mm
- Basal view
  - ■ External nasal valve (lower lateral cartilage, columella and sill)
  - ■ Septum: Caudal dislocation
  - ■ Bulbosity: Excessive cartilage width
  - ■ Columella: Height, retraction

    Figure 5.3: Nasal profile and measurements/angles.

3. Palpation:
   - – Skin thickness, irregularity, nodules
   - – Tip support, recoil

   - Dynamic assessment
     - Cottle's manoeuvre: Internal nasal valve collapse
     - Exaggerated inspiration: External nasal valve collapse
     - Cold spatula test: Crude assessment of nasal flow
4. Anterior rhinoscopy:
   - Mucosal assessment: Septum, turbinates (hypertrophy), telangiectasia, ulceration, congestion
   - Structural: Polyps, masses, tumours, septal assessment
5. Nasendoscopy:
   - Flexible or rigid: Detailed assessment of internal anatomy including middle meatus and PNS in the context of a unilateral middle ear effusion
6. Conclusion:
   - Thank the patient and ask if they have any questions
   - Relay to the examiner that you would complete your examination by undertaking:
     - A full head and neck examination for adenopathy (eschelon nodes level II–III for anterior and posterior nose, II–V for PNS)
     - Oral cavity: Palatal examination, OAF
     - Otoscopy: >40% PNS masses present with middle ear effusion

Head and Neck

1. Introduction:
   - Introduce yourself by name and role
   - Confirm the patient's details (name and date of birth)
   - Explain the steps of examination you are planning to undertake
   - Empower the patient to ask questions or stop you at any time
   - Confirm that the patient consents for you to proceed
2. General inspection: Frontal and lateral views
   - Voice assessment: Volume, hoarseness, clarity, slurring
   - Skin assessment: Radiotherapy changes, scars (see "Head and Neck" chapter for reference)
   - Stomal assessment: Tracheostomy/laryngectomy, remove HME/base plate to view patency, assess TOF
   - Masses: Adenopathy, goitre or other midline masses (dynamic assessment with tongue protrusion and swallowing)
   - Oral cavity and oropharynx with aid of a tongue depressor
3. Palpation:
   - Skin: Firm post radiotherapy changes
   - Lymphadenopathy: Palpate all levels including occiput, incorporating salivary glands (ballot SMG) (Figure 5.4)

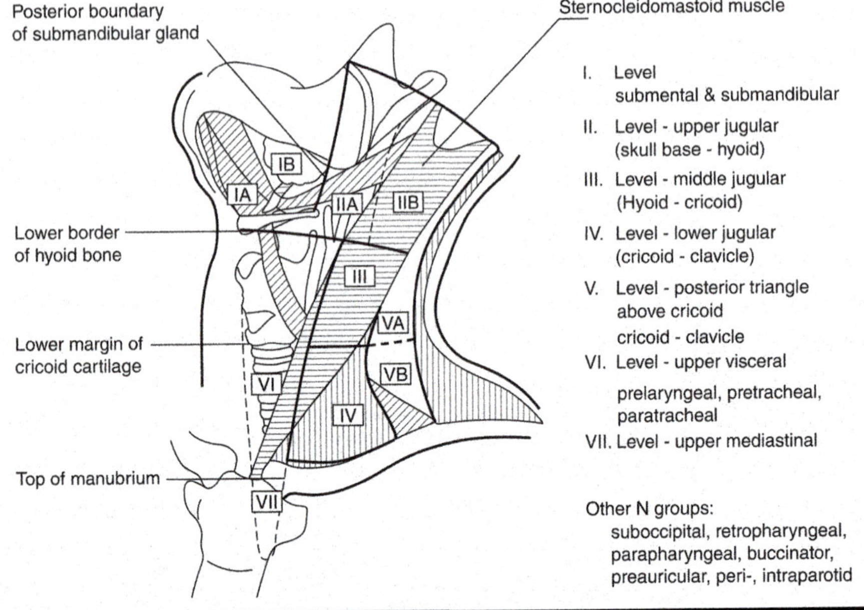

Figure 5.4 Nodal levels and boundaries.

        - Size, texture, pain, irregularity, fixation
    - Thyroid: Normal or enlarged (diffuse, solitary, multinodular, tender)
    - Trachea: Assess for deviation
4. Percussion: To assess for retrosternal extension
5. Auscultation: Thyroid bruit (increased vascularity associated with hyperdynamic circulation)
6. Conclusion:
    - Thank the patient and ask if they have any questions
    - Relay to the examiner that you would complete your examination by:
        - Assessing for further scars: Arm (right forearm, delto-pectoral), chest (pectoralis major), abdomen (jejunal), leg (anterolateral thigh, gracilis)
        - Cranial nerve examination (facial nerve assessment)
        - Flexible nasendoscopy to assess for potential sites of a primary malignancy
        - Thyroid status assessment:
            - Eyes: Proptosis/exophthalmos, ophthalmoplegia
            - Heart: Pulse (rate and regularity), murmur
            - Hands: Pallor, temperature, tremor, texture of skin
            - Legs: Proximal myopathy, reflexes, pre-tibial myxoedema, thyroid acropachy

Level	*Description*	*Boundaries*
1a	**Submental**	Symphysis of mandible, body of hyoid, AB of digastric muscles
1b	**Submandibular**	Body of mandible, PB and AB of digastric muscle, stylohyoid muscle
2a	**Upper Jugular**	Skull base, inf border of hyoid, stylohyoid muscle, vertical plane defined by spinal accessory nerve
2b		Skull base, inf body of hyoid, vertical plane defined by spinal accessory nerve, lateral border of SCM muscle
3	**Middle Jugular**	Inf border of hyoid, inf border of cricoid, lateral border of the sternohyoid muscle, lateral border of the SCM muscle
4	**Lower Jugular**	Inf border of cricoid, clavicle, lateral border of sternohyoid muscle, lateral border of SCM muscle
5	**Posterior Triangle**	Anterior border of trapezius muscle, clavicle and posterior border of SCM muscle 5a above horizontal plane of anterior cricoid arch, Vb below this plane
6	**Anterior Compartment**	Hyoid, suprasternal notch, CCA laterally
7	**Mediastinal**	Suprasternal notch, innominate artery, sternum, trachea, oesophagus, prevertebral fascia

Cranial Nerves

1. Introduction:
   - Introduce yourself by name and role
   - Confirm the patient's details (name and date of birth)
   - Explain the steps of examination you are planning to undertake
   - Empower the patient to ask questions or stop you at any time
   - Confirm that the patient consents for you to proceed

2. Examination:
   - I: Olfactory
     - Changes in smell
     - Can formally assess with UPSIT
   - II: Optic
     - Visual acuity: Snellen chart
     - Visual fields: All four quadrants whilst covering contralateral eye
     - Reflexes: Pupillary light reflex, accommodation reflex, RAPD
     - Colour: Ishihara chart
     - Fundoscopy
   - III, IV, VI: Oculomotor, trochlear, abducens: Eye movements
     - III palsy: Ptosis (levator palpebrae superioris), downward and outward eye (lateral rectus exerts control over paralysed medial rectus, as well as superior oblique over the inferior, superior rectus, inferior oblique)
     - IV palsy: Diplopia with inferomedial gaze
     - VI palsy: Failure of abduction
   - V: Trigeminal
     - Sensory: V1, V2 and V3 as well as sensation to anterior 2/3 of tongue
       - Corneal reflex
     - Motor: Tensor tympani. Muscles of mastication
       - Medial and lateral pterygoid, temporalis, masseter. Jaw deviates to site of lesion
   - VII: Facial
     - Sensory: Taste to anterior 2/3 of tongue via chorda tympani
     - Motor: Muscles of facial expression, stapedius, posterior belly of digastric
   - VIII: Vestibulocochlear
     - Hearing: Free field testing, tuning forks, pure tone audiometry
     - Vestibular: Dix-Hallpike manoeuvre, Unterberger test
   - IX: Glossopharyngeal
     - Sensory: Taste and sensation to posterior 1/3 of tongue
     - Motor: Stylopharyngeus muscle, gag reflex
   - X: Vagus
     - Sensory: External ear
     - Motor:
       - Voice (recurrent laryngeal nerve)
       - Soft palate/uvula deviation (away from lesion)
       - Gag reflex
       - Swallowing (pharyngeal constrictors)
   - XI: Accessory: Shrug shoulders (trapezius) and turn head (sternocleidomastoid)

- XII: Hypoglossal
  - Tongue wasting, fasciculations
  - Protrusion of tongue (deviation towards site of lesion)

3C's of papilloedema

- Cupping (large cup: Disc ratio >0.5)
- Colour (pale)
- Contour (loss)

Chapter 6

Communication Stations

Wai Sum Cho, Anna Slovick, Jameel Muzaffar and Adnan Darr

Contents

DOI: 10.1201/9781003247098-6

Introduction

The communication skills station is set up to mimic what you do in your day-to-day job. The station lasts 20 minutes and your interaction is with an actor/actress, and accounts for 10% of your overall mark for part B. You will be given some background information and will be asked if you understand the scenario by your examiners before you start. It is useful to note that there is ample time allocated for this station so remember to take your time during the consultation.

In general, the communication skills station is separated into two to three parts. The first part involves history taking, gathering of information and formulating further investigations. The second part is likely to involve an explanation of the results of the investigations, diagnosis and consenting for any intervention. There might be a third part of the consultation, which may involve discussion about complications following surgery.

During the scenario, you will be assessed in the way you conduct the consultation, pick up on any non-verbal cues and ability to incorporate all the information given to formulate a sensible management plan. You will be observed on how you explain your diagnosis to the patient, avoiding jargons.

Whilst the aim of the communications part of the exam is not to assess your knowledge, there will be some knowledge component incorporated during the consenting process and answering any questions the patient has. Remember to treat the station just like how you approach your consultation during your day-to-day work. Be relaxed, introduce yourself and confirm patient details before proceeding with your consultation.

Important points to note for this station include taking into account the patient's occupation and hobbies. When explaining the diagnosis, utilise drawings/illustrations (if applicable), remember to sign post and involve other members of the team (specialist nurses, speech and language therapist). Always ensure time to complete the consultation by offering a point of contact or written information sheets/websites, where relevant, and ensuring the patient has no additional ideas, concerns or expectations. There may be a hidden agenda from the patient's point of view to be addressed, such as a patient with tinnitus being worried about having a brain tumour.

Scenario 1: The Noisy Baby

An ex-28-week premature baby, now 15-month-old, corrected was brought to you in clinic with noisy breathing.

Part 1:

- History taking from parent and recommended investigations
- Points to cover:
  - Nature and duration of noisy breathing, cyanotic episodes, feeding

  - Any previous intubation (number and duration)
  - Any diagnosed airway problems
  - Impact of breathing problems on baby such as growth
  - Check the red book
- You decide that the baby requires a diagnostic laryngotracheobronchoscopy. Please go through the procedure and obtain consent
- Additional points to cover:
  - To also consent for possibility of treating any potential pathology seen such as balloon dilatation or aryepiglottoplasty for subglottic stenosis or laryngomalacia
  - Discuss the small possibility of intensive care stay post procedure

Part 2:

- You diagnosed subglottic stenosis with 60% narrowing of the airway. You decided to perform balloon dilatation to improve the airway. Unfortunately following the procedure, there was significant oedema and the baby had to be kept intubated. Speak to the parents about your diagnosis and further management plan
- Points to cover:
  - Oedema is expected and likely to be temporary
  - Inform the potential need for further procedures in the future
  - Discuss the possibility of requiring tracheostomy or surgical procedure to the airway such as a cricoid split. They may need to be referred to a tertiary centre
- Parental concerns: Parents are worried about the need for a tracheostomy and the long-term care/impact having seen another child requiring one during previous admission

Scenario 2: A Regurgitating Patient

A 55-year-old male presents to you in outpatients with a 6-month history of food regurgitation, dysphagia and halitosis.

Part 1:

- Initial consultation of patient and investigations
- Points to cover:
  - Red flag symptoms such as referred otalgia, odynophagia, weight loss
  - Ask about recurrent chest infections
  - Smoking and alcohol history
  - Impact on quality of life

Part 2:

- You decided to request a barium swallow and it shows a pharyngeal pouch about 1 vertebral body in size. Explain your diagnosis to the patient, further management plan and consent for any procedure you decide to do
- Points to cover:
  - Try using illustrations to explain a pharyngeal pouch to the patient
  - Explain treatment options including conservative management, endoscopic stapling and external approach
  - Remember to also consent for recurrence, hoarse voice, unable to perform procedure due to access problems and perforation requiring prolonged inpatient stay and a nasogastric feeding tube

Part 3:

- During the operation, access was very difficult and you were unable to proceed with stapling of the pouch. You were worried about a perforation and decided to insert a nasogastric feeding tube and keep the patient nil by mouth for 5 days. Explain to the patient your operative findings and further management plan
- During the consultation, you found that the patient is refusing to stay in hospital for 5 days as he is the main carer for his son who has learning disability
- Points to cover:
  - Explain about difficulty with access and concern about perforation
  - Address patient's concern: Explore if son is known to learning disability team/have any support packages at home
  - Allow opportunity for patient to arrange care at home
  - Discuss potential alternatives such as a water-soluble contrast swallow or CT scan with oral contrast to assess for any leak of which, if clear, may be able to be discharged

Scenario 3: A Lumpy Neck

A 60-year-old female presents to you at the head and neck clinic with a 3-year history of enlarging midline neck mass.

Part 1:

- Initial consultation and examination
- Examination subsequently showed a 5 × 4 cm likely thyroid neck mass
- Points to cover:
  - Head and neck history including red flag symptoms such as pain, weight loss
  - Ask about compressive symptoms and impact on quality of life (patient enjoys long walks)
  - Thyroid status

- History of radiation exposure or family history of thyroid cancer
- Arrange further investigations

Part 2:

- Ultrasound scan shows U2 multinodular goitre with no retrosternal extension and no lymphadenopathy. Thyroid function tests were within normal limits. The patient reports difficulty with exertion and lying flat. You decide that the patient requires total thyroidectomy. Explain the scan results and take consent
- Points to cover:
  - Mass is non-cancerous
  - Need for long-term thyroid supplementation
  - During consenting process also discuss possibility of long-term calcium replacements, hoarse voice, bilateral vocal cord palsy and tracheostomy

Part 3:

- Following surgery, the patient developed stridor and significant respiratory distress in recovery. Flexible nasendoscopy showed bilateral vocal cord palsy. You decided to perform a tracheostomy and insertion of a nasogastric feeding tube. Explain your surgical findings and management plan to the family members
- Points to cover:
  - Bilateral vocal cord palsy may be temporary or permanent
  - Tracheostomy likely temporary but may be permanent depending on recovery, swallow and aspiration risk
  - Discuss about swallowing assessments and potentially removal of feeding tube
  - Discuss possibility of going home with tracheostomy but dependent of recovery and support available for patient and family from airway nurse specialist

Scenario 4: Facial Asymmetry

A 46-year-old male, previously treated for Bell's palsy at your hospital's emergency department a year ago, now presents to your clinic with an enlarging parotid mass on the same side.

Part 1:

- Initial consultation and examination
- Examination showed a right 3 × 2 cm firm parotid mass with possible ipsilateral lymphadenopathy. The patient had a grade 6 facial weakness
- Points to cover:
  - Take history about the parotid swelling going through other potential causes
  - Assess for red flag signs

  - Assess facial function, ask if it was a gradual deterioration and if there has been any recovery
  - Smoking and alcohol history
  - If patient asks, explain suspicious of cancer and require further investigations which you will arrange urgently
  - Give advice about eye care and contact ophthalmology if patient develops red eye/pain

Part 2:

- Cytology showed adenoid cystic carcinoma and imaging confirmed neck level 2 lymphadenopathy but no distant metastasis. The case has been discussed at the MDT meeting and total parotidectomy, neck dissection, facial nerve sacrifice and reconstruction are recommended. The patient will also require postoperative radiotherapy. Explain to the patient the results and recommended treatment
- In this part, the patient will be very upset that the diagnosis has been missed. He will ask if his prognosis is now worse
- Points to cover:
  - Set the scene, offer patient's partner/family member to sit in, including a head and neck specialist nurse
  - Apologise to the patient for the late diagnosis
  - Avoid criticising your colleagues at the emergency department
  - Explain that an incident form has been completed and further investigation would be performed by the hospital
  - You would take the initiative to change the hospital's pathway for patients presenting with facial palsy so they would be assessed by ENT if there is no recovery within a certain period to ensure similar situation would not happen again
  - Offer contact number for PALS
  - Be honest with the patient, prognosis may be worse due to the delay in diagnosis
  - Offer a date for surgery and give contact number of secretary and head and neck nurse specialist as point of contact for any queries or problems

Scenario 5: A Worrying Neck Mass

A 72-year-old female presents with a rapidly enlarging midline neck mass and a hoarse voice.

Part 1:

- Initial consultation and examination

- Examination showed a firm midline neck mass with ill-defined edges. Flexible nasendoscopy demonstrated right vocal cord palsy
- Points to cover:
  - If asked, share with patient suspicion that it may be cancer
  - Arrange urgent investigations such as ultrasound guided aspiration for cytology and CT scan

Part 2:

- Cytology results were consistent with anaplastic thyroid cancer and CT scan showed a large infiltrative mass encasing the right carotid artery, multiple cervical lymphadenopathy and likely lung metastasis. The tumour is now also fungating through the skin. The case has been discussed at the MDT and best supportive care has been recommended. You now need to inform the patient of the diagnosis and management plan
- Points to cover:
  - Adopt the **SPIKES** algorithm when breaking bad news:
    - **S**etting (relatives to sit in, specialist nurse)
    - **P**erception (determine how much the patient already knows)
    - **I**nvitation (explore if the patient would like to know all the details about the diagnosis)
    - **K**nowledge (give small amounts of information at a time and check patient understanding, allowing time to ask questions)
    - **E**mpathy (give patient opportunity to express their feelings, provide box of tissues)
    - **S**ummary (summarise the diagnosis and management plan, allow patient time to ask questions)
  - Inform the patient that there are no curative options
  - Discuss palliative treatments/input from the palliative care team to assist with pain and symptom control
  - Discuss option of palliative radiotherapy to help with the fungating tumour or pain symptoms
  - If the patient gets breathless in the future, discuss potential option of palliative tracheostomy which can help with breathing but has the disadvantages of further tumour infiltration, skin breakdown and requiring tracheostomy care
  - Provide opportunity for further appointment

Scenario 6: Voice Change

A 65-year-old male smoker presents to you at a 2-week wait clinic with an 8-week history of hoarse voice.

Part 1:

- Initial consultation
- Examination subsequently revealed a lesion on the middle third of the right true vocal cord with normal mobility. Neck examination was normal
- Points to cover:
  - Head and neck history including red flag symptoms such as referred otalgia, odynophagia, weight loss
  - Smoking and alcohol history
  - Occupation and hobbies: Patient sings in a church choir
  - Consent for microlaryngoscopy and biopsy
  - Discuss smoking cessation

Part 2:

- Histology results show squamous cell carcinoma and following imaging the staging is T1aN0M0. The case has been discussed at the MDT and it was decided that both transoral laser resection and radiotherapy are suitable treatment options. Inform patient of the diagnosis and further management plan
- Points to cover:
  - Offer patient to have partner/friend to sit in the consultation in attendance with a head and neck specialist nurse
  - Break bad news that it is cancer but stress that cancer is caught early and prognosis is very good
  - Discuss treatment options: Surgery (transoral laser) vs radiotherapy
  - The patient opted for transoral laser surgery to treat her cancer, obtain consent for the procedure

Part 3:

- The surgery went very well and histology showed complete excision of the tumour. This is your follow up appointment to discuss histology results
- The patient was very upset, as she was unable to sing and was expecting her voice to be back to normal. Flexible nasendoscopy was unremarkable
- Points to cover:
  - Explain to the patient that the cancer has safely been removed and no further treatment is required other than regular follow-up
  - Ensure the patient has realistic expectations with regard to her voice quality following surgery, reassure that voice should get better but might not be back to normal
  - Discuss voice rest, acid reflux treatment and input from SALT team
  - Provide contact for PALS and second opinion if the patient remains unhappy and would like to make a formal complaint

Scenario 7: The Snoring Child

A 5-year-old girl was brought to your clinic due to a history of snoring.

Part 1:

- Initial consultation and examination
- Examination showed grade 4 tonsils and a snotty nose
- Points to cover:
  - Establish if there is a history of sleep apnoea, duration, cyanotic episodes and any nasal obstruction
  - Ask if there is a video of the child sleeping
  - Decide if there is also a history of recurrent tonsillitis
  - Ask about impact on quality of life and behaviour

Part 2:

- Sleep study results show evidence of moderate sleep apnoea. You decide to offer adenotonsillectomy due to a history of recurrent tonsillitis as well. Please obtain consent from the parents
- Points to cover:
  - Discuss aim of surgery and potential complications including bleeding (parents would then share that they are Jehovah's witnesses and decline all blood products in the event that any would be needed)
  - Be respectful of the family's religious beliefs
  - Consider different techniques such as coblation intracapsular tonsillectomy to reduce the risk of postoperative bleeding but balance with the risk of tonsillar regrowth and continue to suffer from tonsillitis
  - To liaise with anaesthetic colleague including preoperative work up to assess baseline blood count

Part 3:

- You decided to perform adenotonsillectomy which went uneventfully. Unfortunately, the child attended the emergency department 8 days later with a large post tonsillectomy bleed and signs of grade 4 hypovolemic shock. As the on-call consultant, please speak to the family about your management plan
- Points to cover:
  - Establish with the family the severity of the situation
  - Obtain consent for surgery to arrest the bleeding
  - Explain the need for blood transfusion and importance to save the child's life
  - Offer to obtain a second opinion and a haematologist to see if they agree with your assessment and if there are any alternatives

- As this is an emergency situation, if parents continue to decline blood transfusion, discuss that in the best interest of the child, you have a duty to intervene to save the child's life – before proceeding, obtain a second opinion ± emergency Trust legal advice. Healthcare professionals may face criminal prosecution if a child comes to harm because treatment was withheld

GMC Good Medical Practice:

In an emergency, you can provide treatment that is immediately necessary to save life or prevent deterioration in health without consent or, in exceptional circumstances, against the wishes of a person with parental responsibility.

Scenario 8: A Discharging Ear

A 38-year-old male presents to you in the clinic with a 3-month history of right-sided hearing loss and ear discharge.

Part 1:

- Initial consultation and examination
- Examination showed attic defect with granulation tissue
- Audiogram showed a 50 dB right-sided conductive hearing loss
- Points to cover:
  - Obtain otology history
  - Remember to ask about occupation and any hobbies
  - Discuss with the patient that you suspect a cholesteatoma and would like to further investigate and plan further management by performing a CT scan

Part 2:

- Following a CT scan, you diagnose a cholesteatoma and would like to perform a combined approach tympanomastoidectomy. Explain the diagnosis and obtain consent
- Points to cover:
  - Explain the diagnosis, try to utilise illustrations to explain cholesteatoma and potential complications i.e. retraction pocket causing abnormal migration of keratin and collection of debris causing local erosion and persistent infection
  - Explain your surgical approach and take consent (bleeding, infection, tinnitus, dizziness, worsen hearing including dead ear, taste change, facial palsy [temporary/permanent], CSF leak leading to meningitis, recurrence)

- Discuss possibility of performing ossiculoplasty at the same time
- Discuss the role of MR DWI as part of follow up or second look a year later

Part 3:

- You performed the surgery, which was uneventful and you planned to perform an MR DWI in 1 yr. Due to persistent discharging ear following surgery, you decided to perform an early second look surgery at 6 months. During the operation, you found a retained cotton wool ball and no cholesteatoma. Explain to the patient about your operation findings
- Points to cover:
  - Be honest with the patient and apologise for the retained foreign body, which is likely to be the cause of the infection
  - Inform the patient that this is a severe event and you are taking this very seriously
  - An incident form has been completed and further investigation would be performed to assess how this occurred and steps implemented so it wouldn't happen again
  - Offer to formalise "duty of candor" to patient by providing update on the outcome of the investigation by writing
  - Offer contact number for PALS

Scenario 9: The Young Patient with Hearing Loss

A 25-year-old female presents to you in outpatients with a history of hearing loss.

Part 1:

- Initial consultation and examination
- Points to cover:
  - Obtain otology history (tinnitus, dizziness, balance disturbance, discharge, otalgia)
  - Determine if hearing loss is unilateral/bilateral, progressive, previous head injuries
  - Establish occupation, hobbies, loud noise exposure and impact on quality of life
  - Does the patient already use hearing aids?
  - Past medical history such as previous surgeries, hypothyroidism, renal disease
  - Neonatal history/infections, NICU stay, ototoxic drug use
  - Family history of hearing loss

Part 2:

- Examination was unremarkable
- Audiogram showed bilateral, symmetrical hearing loss at 60 dB, type A tympanometry and aided AB word score of 75%

  During the consultation, the patient will be pushing for cochlear implants

- Points to cover:
  - Explain that patient has significant hearing loss
  - Offer investigations such as blood tests to assess for an autoimmune cause and MRI scan to assess for pathologies such as enlarged vestibular aqueduct syndrome
  - Establish if the patient uses hearing aids and if she has found it beneficial – may benefit from seeing audiologist for hearing aid optimisation and hearing therapy
  - Offer tinnitus therapy
  - Explore what the patient understands about cochlear implants
  - Explain that cochlear implant does not offer natural hearing
  - At current level, based on current evidence and NICE guidelines, the patient is more likely to benefit from optimisation of current hearing and hearing aids than with cochlear implantation
  - Explain that hearing is likely to get worse over time and can be reassessed for cochlear implantation in the future if she finds her hearing is deteriorating

Scenario 10: Do I Have a Brain Tumour?

You are called by your SHO to review a 40-year-old male in the emergency clinic with right-sided acute hearing loss.

Part 1:

- Initial consultation and examination
- Points to cover:
  - Obtain otology history and history of trauma
  - Establish if it was a sudden onset hearing loss
  - Assess for potential cranial nerve deficit such as double vision, facial numbness, facial twitching/weakness (sudden enlargement of cystic VS)
  - Also ask about past medical history, specifically history of autoimmune disease
  - Obtain a drug history focusing on any ototoxic medications
  - Ask about the patient's occupation – the patient works on the railway

Part 2:

- Examination was normal and the audiogram showed a profound right-sided sensorineural hearing loss. You decide that the patient requires a course of oral prednisolone. Explain the condition to the patient and your management plan
- Points to cover:
  - Explain likely aetiology of sudden sensorineural hearing loss and need for an MRI scan
  - Discuss aim of treatment and potential side effects
  - Explore potential contraindications for systemic steroid treatment in the patient (i.e. GI bleed, previous psychosis on steroids)
  - Discuss likely prognosis
  - Advise the patient to inform work as the patient now has single-sided deafness which might impact on his work on the railway

Part 3:

- You see the patient 4 months later and the audiogram remains unchanged. His MRI scan is unremarkable
- Points to cover:
  - Approach this part of the station similar to breaking bad news as his hearing is unlikely to recover
  - Explore impact on quality of life and work
  - Offer tinnitus therapy (if applicable)
  - Discuss hearing rehabilitation options and their limitations such as CROS hearing aid and bone conduction hearing aid
  - Discuss long-term difficulty with sound localisation

Scenario 11: What's That Ringing?

In outpatients, you prepare to review a new referral. The GP letter states "I would be grateful for your assessment of Mrs Brown, a 65 year old female who complains of ringing in her left ear."

Part 1:

- Initial consultation and examination
- Points to cover:
  - Obtain otology history, including history of noise exposure, trauma, ototoxic medication and family history
  - Delve deeper into subjective complaints (unilateral/bilateral/pulsatile/musical), when it started, how long present for, how troublesome

- Ideas, concerns and expectations i.e. is this a brain tumour?
- Otoscopic/otoendoscopic examination plus pure tone audiogram

Part 2:

- Mrs Brown reports left unilateral non-pulsatile, intermittent tinnitus. Clinical Examination was normal and the audiogram showed a symmetrical high-frequency sensorineural hearing loss in keeping with her age. Explain the condition to the patient and your management plan
- Points to cover:
  - Explain likely aetiology of tinnitus (with or without hearing loss) and need for an MRI scan with approximate rate of pathology (roughly 1:100)
  - Discuss treatment options (hearing aid/tinnitus therapy)
  - Potential use of masking devices
  - Discuss likely prognosis
  - Support groups i.e. British Tinnitus Association

Part 3:

- 6 months later, Mrs Brown is rereferred as her symptoms have become bilateral. She declined referral for hearing aid or tinnitus therapy. Her MRI scan was unremarkable and clinical examination and PTA are unchanged
- Points to cover:
  - Gently revisit the previous options (Hearing aid, tinnitus therapy)
  - Explore impact on quality of life and work
  - Discuss long-term habituation

Scenario 12: The Challenging Family

You are the on-call consultant when the registrar calls you to see a 70-year-old female currently in ED resus with stridor. Flexible nasendoscopy reveals a glottic tumour and bilateral vocal cord palsy and the decision is made to go to theatre for a tracheostomy under local anaesthetic. After the case, the patient asks you to explain the situation to their son and daughter, who have now arrived at the hospital.

Part 1:

- Initial discussion
- Points to cover:
  - Introduce yourself, clarify who they are
  - Explore what they already know and understand
  - Explain the likely diagnosis, further workup and potential treatment options

Part 2:

- The patient stays in hospital and undergoes cross sectional imaging showing widely disseminated disease. Histology from the biopsy you took at the time of tracheostomy shows SCC. The MDT feels that the best supportive care, with or without palliative chemotherapy, would be most appropriate. You meet the patient with their two adult children in outpatients
- Points to cover:
  - Explain the results to the patient, including the rationale for potentially palliative treatment and the difference from curative intent
  - One of the children is very angry about this and wants full active treatment. The other child and the parent are understanding of the situation

Part 3:

- Three months later, the patient is readmitted with worsening pain. The nursing staff ask you to discuss resuscitation status with the patient
- Points to cover:
  - Explain likely futility of CPR in patients with advanced disease
  - Explore patient views
  - Explain what happens during CPR
  - The patient asks you not to tell their children – what should you do?

Scenario 13: The Anosmic Patient

You are asked to review a patient in outpatient clinic who has previously been diagnosed with chronic rhinosinusitis with polyposis. She has been trialled on multiple topical therapies for many years, including oral steroids on three occasions in the past 12 months. A CT was requested, which demonstrates diffuse polyposis throughout all sinuses.

Part 1:

- Points to cover:
  - Summarises reasons for attendance and understanding
  - Discusses findings of CT scan, and offers to show images if present
  - Discusses role of surgery, but advises that recurrence rates are high
  - Discusses risks associated with surgery: GA, pain, infection, bleeding, smell/taste disturbances, recurrence, orbital injury (1:3000), visual disturbance (including blindness), CSF leak (1:1000), COVID risk

Part 2:

- Patient agrees to surgery and presents to outpatients clinic 12-weeks later. Procedure was undertaken by a colleague, who documented an intra-operative lamina breach. Patient has ongoing diplopia. Was adamant nobody discussed complication pre or post operatively
- Points to cover:
  - Apologises and claims accountability for complication, even if complication had been previously discussed. Offers to discuss consenting process within department to ensure patient understanding in future
  - Assesses impact of complication on day-to-day life: Explores occupation (patient is a secretary at a legal firm and cannot fulfil duties at present)
  - Advises that there may be an improvement, but does not commit to timing
  - Offers to contact ophthalmology team urgently to expedite assessment
  - Provides contact details for PALS for formal complaint who will deal with any further action
  - Provides own contact details to patient if there are any further questions, but also offers a second opinion or transfer of care depending on relationship during encounter

Scenario 14: Awkward Conversations

You are asked by a GP to review a 45-year-old male with his wife, who has presented with a 2-month history of a large left level 2 neck node.

Part 1:

- Initial consultation of patient, examination and investigations
- Points to cover:
  - History of presenting complaint
  - Red flag symptoms: Otalgia, odynophagia, dyspnoea, dysphonia and weight loss
  - Smoking and alcohol history

Part 2:

- Oropharyngeal examination shows an ulcerated left tonsil. With the exception of the examined node, the remainder of the examination including nasendoscopy is unremarkable
- Points to cover:
  - Relays findings to patient and partner
  - Requests USS + FNAC, as well as MRI neck and CT thorax
  - Can offer to biopsy in clinic as obvious lesion, but GA biopsy also sufficient plan

Part 3:

- Results of biopsies and USS/FNAC show a T3N2aM0 P16 +ve oropharyngeal SCC. The MDT recommends chemoradiotherapy
- Points to cover:
  - Initial discussion about previous appointments, investigations and understanding
  - Pauses between information delivered
  - Relays findings of histology as well as radiology discussed at the MDT
  - Explains the nature of the cancer (HPV), and likely better outcomes in young non-smoking patients compared to non-HPV smokers
  - Offers to further appointments to discuss any further concerns
  - Arranges a session with head and neck nurse specialists to answer any potential questions

Part 4:

- The patient's partner asks to speak to you alone after the consultation. She states that she knows a friend who had a similar cancer and was told that it was a sexually transmitted disease. She asks "is my partner cheating on me?"
- Points to cover:
  - Discusses HPV in general, rather than in context of patient, as confidentiality still needs to be maintained
  - Explains that HPV is a viral infection, and one mode of spread is sexual contact
  - Explains that virus may remain dormant for many years, prior to presentation as a malignancy
  - Advises that it is important now to focus on the treatment, and reassures partner with regard to overall prognosis

Scenario 15: A Complicated Tonsillitis

You are asked to review a 12-year-old child on your round who came in overnight with a suspected quinsy. She had been admitted by the SHO following discussion with the registrar. On the ward round, you see a stridulous child with torticollis and note an associated neck swelling. You stabilise her with adrenaline nebulisers and IV steroids. A CT is performed which confirms your suspicion of a parapharyngeal abscess. You look at the drug chart and none of the appropriate antibiotics or steroids had been prescribed since admission. The father would like to speak to you.

Part 1:

- Please explain what you would tell the father
- Points to cover:
  - History, examination findings and diagnosis
  - Explains the next steps for management of the condition
  - Apologises that this had not been suspected by the admitting Dr and that the appropriate treatment was not given, in accordance with duty of candor
  - Explains that this will be discussed in the next departmental meeting and discussed with the team concerned

Part 2:

- A decision is made to take the child to theatre. Please kindly take consent from the father
- Points to cover:
  - Discusses open vs closed drainage
  - Includes the possible need for tracheostomy, NG tube insertion or paediatric intensive care stay following operation

Scenario 16: Duty of Care and Support

A 70-year-old male smoker presents with progressive dysphagia, hoarse voice and weight loss. He is admitted to hospital for investigation for a suspected malignancy and management of his malnutrition. As the consultant on the ward round, it is brought to your attention by the nurse that the patient is complaining of left calf tenderness and swelling. Investigations reveal a Deep Vein Thrombosis (DVT). You notice that DVT prophylaxis was not written up by the admitting doctor. His daughter is visiting and wants to speak with you.

Part 1:

- Please explain the sequence of events to his concerned daughter
  - Establishes a rapport with his daughter, ensuring her understanding of the situation is sought
  - Summarises the history, examination findings and investigations to date
  - Explains the likely diagnosis of DVT and the next steps for management of the condition
  - Apologises that the appropriate prophylactic treatment was not given, in accordance with duty of candor
  - Explains that an incident form will be completed, that this will be discussed in the next departmental meeting and directly discussed with the doctors concerned in order to minimise recurrence

Part 2:

- You are taken into the office by the ward manager who has raised concerns about a junior doctor, who is "persistently" ignoring venous thromboembolism assessments, and failing to prescribe the relevant treatment. On further inspection, it appears that this was the same junior doctor involved in the care of the aforementioned patient. You request a face-to-face meeting with the CT1 doctor to discuss the matter
- Points to cover:
  - Ensure an empathetic approach is maintained as there could be a variety of reasons for omission
  - Ask about general experience within the department and any areas of concerns they may have

Part 3:

- Doctor explains that part of the reason there have been lapses in concentration is due to recent illness at home, and he is the sole carer of his mother who suffers with dementia
- Points to cover:
  - Continue to approach situation in an empathetic manner, asking about any ways in which the department may assist, for example change in shift patterns, change in on call rota for the foreseeable future
  - Offer educational resources (online) in order to address any knowledge deficits that may have developed
  - Offer to contact both educational supervisor and the Training Programme Director in order to ensure adequate support for the trainee

Scenario 17: Illicit Substance Use

A 23-year-old male banker is referred to you by his GP with profuse nasal crusting and a suspected septal perforation.

Part 1:

- Please take an appropriate history and explain what examination you might like to perform
- Points to cover:
  - Identify potential causes of perforation in history: Trauma, surgery, systemic symptoms (vasculitis), recreational drug use, medications (steroids, decongestants)
  - Symptoms and impact: May be asymptomatic, but whistling may be troublesome, particularly in face-to-face roles

Part 2:

- Examination reveals a large septal perforation with friable mucosa and no ulceration. A saddle nose deformity is also noted
- Please explain the next steps to the patient in terms of investigation
- Points to cover:
  - Blood tests
  - Urinalysis
  - Chest X-ray
  - Possible need for a biopsy depending on the results of the blood tests

Part 3:

- cANCA is positive with urine positive for cocaine. The patient is keen to have their septal perforation and saddle nose repaired, as does not want his girlfriend to notice his perforation. Please discuss the underlying cause of his septal perforation and the management
- Points to cover:
  - Explains the diagnosis
  - Discusses conservative options, such as saline douching and a prescription of rotating nasal antibacterial creams for the crusting
  - Discusses the need to refrain from further cocaine use if wishing to pursue surgical options
  - Mentions surgical options and risks, ensuring to emphasise that these could only be considered once he has managed to refrain from cocaine use for at least 6–12 months
  - Books clinical photography in the meantime
  - Books a follow-up appointment to assess symptoms, test results and whether he has refrained from cocaine use and to discuss surgical options further including septal button or repair

Scenario 18: Addressing Anxiety

A 60-year-old female has been referred to your clinic with progressive dysphagia over the last year. She has a family history of cancer and is incredibly anxious.

Part 1:

- Please take a history and explain the examination you would like to perform
- Points to cover:
  - Timing and onset of symptoms. Solids/liquids
  - Previous history of head and neck malignancy/treatment (CRT)
  - Other red flag features: Dysphonia, dyspnoea, odynophagia, referred otalgia
  - Smoking/drinking history

Part 2:

- She is found to have a history of fatigue, angular cheilitis, with intermittent dysphagia particularly to solids. She has had no weight loss. Please explain investigations might you like to perform
- Points to cover:
  - Ensures blood tests are performed, including FBC and iron levels
  - Books a barium swallow to check for a web

Part 3:

- She is found to have iron deficiency anaemia with a pharyngo-oesophageal web
- Explain the possible diagnosis and management
- Points to cover:
  - Ensures an explanation of Plummer-Vinson syndrome is given
  - Discusses conservative options such as iron supplements, dietician input like avoidance of tough meat
  - Explains the management of the web such as direct pharyngo-oesophagoscopy ± dilatation ± biopsy
  - Explains the need for follow-up by GP to check for resolution of anaemia and iron studies, after initiation of iron replacement
  - Warns that repeat oesophageal dilations may be required if the symptoms recur
  - Discussed the increased risk of upper oesophageal and hypopharyngeal carcinoma
  - Explores her ideas, concerns and expectations given the family history of cancer

Index

Note: Locators in *italics* represent figures and **bold** indicate tables in the text.